ONCOLOGY SOCIAL WORK PRACTICE IN THE CARE OF BREAST AND OVARIAN CANCER SURVIVORS

ONCOLOGY SOCIAL WORK PRACTICE IN THE CARE OF BREAST AND OVARIAN CANCER SURVIVORS

CINDY DAVIS

Nova Science Publishers, Inc.
New York

For permission to use material from this book please contact us:
Telephone 631-231-7269; Fax 631-231-8175
Web Site: http://www.novapublishers.com

NOTICE TO THE READER

The Publisher has taken reasonable care in the preparation of this book, but makes no expressed or implied warranty of any kind and assumes no responsibility for any errors or omissions. No liability is assumed for incidental or consequential damages in connection with or arising out of information contained in this book. The Publisher shall not be liable for any special, consequential, or exemplary damages resulting, in whole or in part, from the readers' use of, or reliance upon, this material.

Independent verification should be sought for any data, advice or recommendations contained in this book. In addition, no responsibility is assumed by the publisher for any injury and/or damage to persons or property arising from any methods, products, instructions, ideas or otherwise contained in this publication.

This publication is designed to provide accurate and authoritative information with regard to the subject matter covered herein. It is sold with the clear understanding that the Publisher is not engaged in rendering legal or any other professional services. If legal or any other expert assistance is required, the services of a competent person should be sought. FROM A DECLARATION OF PARTICIPANTS JOINTLY ADOPTED BY A COMMITTEE OF THE AMERICAN BAR ASSOCIATION AND A COMMITTEE OF PUBLISHERS.

LIBRARY OF CONGRESS CATALOGING-IN-PUBLICATION DATA

Davis, Cindy.
  Oncology social work practice in the care of breast and ovarian cancer survivors / Cindy Davis.
    p. ; cm.
  Includes bibliographical references and index.
  ISBN 978-1-60692-594-2 (hardcover)
  1. Breast--Cancer--Social aspects. 2. Ovaries--Cancer--Social aspects. 3. Medical social work. I. Title.
  [DNLM: 1. Breast Neoplasms--psychology. 2. Ovarian Neoplasms--psychology. 3. Social Support. 4. Social Work. 5. Survivors--psychology. WP 870 D261o 2009]
  RC280.B8D36283 2009
  362.19699449--dc22
                    2008053594

Published by Nova Science Publishers, Inc. ✦ New York

This book was written in memory of my friend, Brenda Swafford, who taught me so much about the emotional struggles of dying with cancer and leaving young children behind. And, in memory of my children's grandmother, Stella Rollason, whose life was taken by cancer before she got to meet her wonderful grandchildren, Zak and Ali, and see her son, Steve, become an amazing father.

CONTENTS

Preface   ix

Chapter 1   Oncology Social Work   1

Chapter 2   Oncology Social Workers as Patient Navigators   5

Chapter 3   State of Womens' Cancers   9

Chapter 4   Different Faces of Cancer   21

Chapter 5   Health Care in the United States   35

Chapter 6   Financial Burden of Cancer   43

Chapter 7   Practical Concerns   49

Chapter 8   Distress in Cancer Patients   55

Chapter 9   Spirituality   59

Chapter 10   Providing Psychosocial Care: Evidence Based Interventions   65

Chapter 11   Impact on Family and Friends   73

Chapter 12   Advocacy and Cancer   81

Chapter 13   The Changing World of Technology   87

Chapter 14   Challenges and Future Directions for Oncology Social Work   93

Appendix A: Sample Resources for Women with Cancer   99

Appendix B: Sample Resources for Partners   101

Appendix C: Sample Resources for Children   103

Acknowledgments   105

References   107

Index   127

PREFACE

The contemporary women's movement has resulted in important advancements in women's health. Health is no longer viewed as simply a "physical" or "biological" problem; rather, health is viewed as a holistic problem that involves the mind, body, and spirit. Women's cancers are intertwined with our views on femininity, sexuality, and womanhood. Diagnosis of a cancer is often accompanied by a significant physical and emotional toll on the lives of women and their families. It is for these reasons that I decided to write this book exploring how social workers can assist in the psychosocial needs of female cancer survivors and their families.

The information in this book is a combination of reviews of the literature, my personal experience in working with cancer patients, and the stories of women that I have interviewed through my research over the past several years. The women's stories are the foundation of this book and my inspiration. Excerpts from their stories are included throughout this book because it is through their stories that I began to understand the important role that oncology social workers can play in the lives of these women and their families. Each survivor is unique and has her own story to tell. Many of the stories share common themes, but each story has its own unique characteristics. Each survivor plays a number of roles in her story: mother, partner, daughter, caregiver, co-worker, friend, and sister. However, "cancer survivor" is not a familiar role, and this new role is something unexpected which impacts all the other roles one plays in life. Cancer is a complex disease and the implications of a cancer diagnosis are far reaching. This disease touches not only the lives of the women, but also, the lives of partners, children, families, friends, and communities. In order to meet the needs of women cancer survivors, we have to explore all their needs and the needs of family and friends who are impacted by this disease.

Chapter 1

ONCOLOGY SOCIAL WORK

"Social workers have knowledge of resources to hook patients up with what they really need."

WHAT IS AN ONCOLOGY SOCIAL WORKER?

According to the Association of Oncology Social Workers (AOSW), oncology social workers are trained clinical social workers who provide services to address the psychosocial needs of survivors, families, and caregivers [1]. Oncology social workers can be found in a variety of settings such as hospitals, cancer treatment centers, cancer organizations, wellness centers, hospices, and advocacy organizations. The goal of the oncology social worker is to enhance the quality of life of the cancer survivor and their family. Oncology social workers should play an integral part as a member of the treatment team and be available to survivors and their families throughout all phases of the cancer experience.

WHY ONCOLOGY SOCIAL WORKERS?

Most health care providers have little time for any patient-related care other than traditional medical care, and few health care providers devote their limited resources to advocate for the needs of patients outside of medical needs [2]. Most physicians, nurses and other key treatment team members have not had formal education or training on how to advocate for their patients or assist them in self-advocacy [2]. Quality cancer care necessitates a multidisciplinary team approach that allows survivors to access experts other than physicians before, during, and after treatment [3]. As one of the largest allied health professions in the U.S., social workers are a primary provider of psychosocial interventions and services intended to facilitate treatment of cancer and other medical conditions, particularly for minority and underserved women.

The oncology social worker is in a unique position to be a key member of the treatment team and play a fundamental role in assisting in the psychosocial care and advocacy role for cancer survivors [4,5]. According to the Association of Oncology Social Work (AOSW), an oncology social worker is the *primary* professional designated to provide psychosocial services to patients, families and significant others confronted with a potential or actual diagnosis of cancer. An oncology social worker generally holds a Master's Degree in Social Work (MSW) from a nationally accredited school of social work, and has had specialized training in cancer care through continuing education, in-service training, and/ or field experience in a medical setting. The scope of oncology social work includes clinical practice, education, administration, and research [1].

> "The social worker provided books for children to help them understand, information on social security, and information for my husband. If the social worker did not have the answer, she would refer me to a place where I could find it. The nurse referred me to the social worker, but the doctor never mentioned the social worker."

Utilizing psychosocial assessments, multidisciplinary teamwork, supportive counseling, case management, and advocacy, oncology social workers help survivors, families and caregivers [1]:

- manage the many crises of the cancer experience
- learn about the social and emotional impact of cancer
- identify and use sources of support
- find resources to assist with particular needs
- advocate for themselves in the health care system and in communities
- achieve access to quality cancer care
- maintain an acceptable quality of life
- arrange desired end of life care
- receive support during bereavement

ONCOLOGY SOCIAL WORKERS VS. NURSE PRACTITIONERS

A nurse practitioner (NP) is an advanced practice nurse who provides health care services similar to that of a physician. According to the American Academy of Nurse Practitioners (AANP), an NP's focus is on care and cure. Like physicians, NPs approach diagnosis and treatment of health problems with an emphasis on disease prevention and health education. While it is true that NPs also offer counsel to patients, their purpose in counseling is to educate patients on the behaviors affecting health and the specific health problems which may affect quality of life [6].

In contrast, oncology social workers offer more in-depth comprehensive psychosocial services and operate from a strengths-focused perspective. When completing a psychosocial assessment with a patient, the social worker will identify the survivor and family strengths and pre-existing support systems, as well as needs for coping effectively with cancer. The issues addressed can range from cancer treatment expectations to spiritual concerns to community resource referrals. After developing mutual goals with the patient and family, an oncology social worker supports them by actively researching, securing, or creating the resources and programs necessary for optimal psychosocial functioning [1].

The oncology social worker also has training in working with underserved and vulnerable populations. Social workers understand the environmental, financial, and political factors that impact the lives of cancer survivors and the devastating toll these factors have on their cancer treatment and survival outcomes in the underserved. The social worker is trained to anticipate, identify, and help patients to overcome barriers within the health care system. Social work was founded on the principles of helping vulnerable populations overcome systemic barriers to services. Nurse practitioners and oncology social workers are both part of an important team to meet the needs of cancer patients.

SOCIAL WORK THEORETICAL FRAMEWORKS

Oncology social workers utilize a variety of theoretical models to support their work, such as the theory of Health Related Quality of Life, Empowerment Theory, and Strengths Perspective.

The theory of *Health Related Quality of Life (HR-QOL)* [7-9] posits that health related quality of life is related to four interconnected domains:

- physical well-being,
- psychological and emotional well-being,
- social well-being, and
- spiritual well-being.

According to this theory, cancer challenges each of the four domains impacting health related quality of life outcomes. Oncology social workers play a fundamental role in this model by identifying and addressing the three domains of psychological/emotional well-being, social well-being, and spiritual well-being as they impact health outcomes for cancer survivors and their families. Although this theoretical model is widely accepted in the health care domain, the psychological, social, and spiritual factors that contribute to health outcomes are often overlooked or undetected by health care professionals [7,10-15]; therefore, these are the key areas that need to be addressed by the oncology social worker.

Empowerment theory acts as an umbrella for social work values and is one of the guiding theories of oncology social work [16]. Empowerment is the process of enhancing the individual's collective skills so they can influence other people and organizations to regain control over their lives [17-19]. Empowerment assumes that individuals are generally best in understanding their own needs, and that it is optimal for individuals to have the greatest possible control in determining various aspects of their health care [5,17,20,21]. The empowerment approach has been embraced by health educators and providers because it acts as a mediating variable between treatment interventions and the desired outcomes [22]. Research has found that women seek internal organizational control and participatory processes that lead to empowerment more than men [23].

The *strengths perspective* focuses on identifying and utilizing a patient's strengths rather than focusing on the problem areas or weaknesses [24]. This perspective is often a unique approach in the medical arena. Medical professionals generally focus on controlling symptoms and reducing negative behaviors; whereas, the strengths perspective focuses on increasing or utilizing positive behaviors. A strengths approach requires a partnership between the patient and the treatment team. Perhaps most important, it requires the social worker to really listen to what the client has to say and probe for the strengths that have helped them through difficult times in the past. Oncology social workers routinely inquire about a survivor's strengths that will assist her and her family in getting through this life crisis. Those strengths are used as building blocks to guide interventions and develop coping strategies. The strengths approach is closely associated with a holistic and wellness approach, which makes social work a unique member of the treatment team in providing these types of services in the cancer setting.

HOW CAN ONCOLOGY SOCIAL WORK OFFSET MEDICAL COSTS?

The value of the oncology social worker to cancer survivors and families should not be underestimated. In addition to lending a different professional perspective to an interdisciplinary health care team, the oncology social worker provides services that impact the survivor's quality of life, quality of care, and cost of care. By effectively assessing and advocating for the psychosocial needs of a client, the oncology social worker can positively impact the cost of cancer care in the following ways [25]:

- increased opportunities for physicians and nurses to care for other patients
- increased patient compliance with medical regimes
- decreased inpatient length of stay
- decreased number of admissions
- decreased use of health care resources along the continuum of care
- increased client satisfaction of care

"It would be wonderful if patients saw a social worker at very beginning of treatment. The social worker can help people get what they need ... like transportation to treatment."

Chapter 2

ONCOLOGY SOCIAL WORKERS AS PATIENT NAVIGATORS

"I didn't know where to turn when I was diagnosed with cancer. The medical system is so complicated, and I didn't understand what the doctors were saying or how to get through the system. It was very stressful for me and my family. I needed someone to help me, but I had nobody."

Patient navigation is a new initiative in health care aimed at reducing disparities by assisting patients in overcoming barriers within the health care system. Minority and medically underserved groups share a disproportionate burden of the disease's mortality rate. In an attempt to combat social barriers to health care and reduce mortality rates among minority and medically underserved women with breast cancer, Dr. Harold Freedman obtained initial funding in the early 1990s from the American Cancer Society (ACS) to implement one of the first patient navigation programs in the nation. The primary responsibility of the navigator was to help breast cancer patients overcome barriers to care [26].

In 2002, the Center for Disease Control (CDC) and the Lance Armstrong Foundation (LAF) developed *A National Action Plan for Cancer Survivorship: African American Priorities*. Stakeholders in the African American community prioritized the survivorship needs in order of importance as follows:

- access to quality care and services;
- education, training, and communication;
- infrastructure, programs and policies; and
- applied research and surveillance.

Within this report, the need for a patient navigator was identified as a top priority within each area of need. This report affirmed that patient navigation programs are essential in promoting diagnosis and treatment understanding, as well as enhancing the delivery of optimum care among African American women [27]. In 2004, a report by the Trans-Health and Human Services Cancer Health Disparities Progress Review Group identified patient navigation programs as a key factor for eliminating health disparities in cancer [28]. Patient navigators can facilitate timely delivery of care, connect survivors to appropriate resources, and provide educational information on survivorship, as well as deal with practical issues related to health insurance and financial issues.

> "I spent all my time trying to deal with insurance, bills, and trying to get to the different appointments. I think it was worse than the treatment. I got so tired of dealing with everything. I was just overwhelmed. It shouldn't be so complicated!"

On June 29, 2005, President Bush signed into law the Patient Navigation Outreach and Chronic Disease Prevention Act (2005) (P.L. 109-18). The Act is a coordinated federal effort to establish standards of practice. The act specifies the following six duties for patient navigators:

1) Act as contacts and coordinators of health care services.
2) Work with community organizations by creating partnerships with patient advocacy groups, charities, health care centers, community hospice centers, other health care providers, or other organizations in the targeted community.
3) Notify individuals of clinical trials and facilitate enrollment of eligible individuals in these trials.
4) Anticipate, identify, and help patients to overcome barriers within the health care system.
5) Coordinate with the relevant health insurance ombudsman programs.
6) Conduct ongoing outreach to health disparity populations.

Although the Patient Navigation Act appears to be a responsive health care initiative, and requires patient navigators to have direct knowledge of the communities they serve, it does not go far enough in establishing standards for quality of care [29]. Dohan and Schrag conducted a review of patient navigation programs and found lack of a standard definition for patient navigators in addition to even greater diversity among patient navigation program components and processes [30]. Patient navigation programs are most commonly implemented in the early phases of screening and diagnosis, but these programs have been implemented at all stages of cancer care (e.g., prevention, screening, treatment, and survival) [30]. There is great inconsistency in who should perform the role of the navigator (e.g., professional or layperson) and the scope of their work. In a review of 11 patient navigation programs, Dohan and Schrag found that seven programs used lay workers while the other four used professionals (nurses or social workers); however, the roles and scope of the navigator varied greatly across programs [30].

Initial research demonstrates that patient navigation is associated with improved outcomes for screening and follow-up, lower clinical stages of presentation, higher levels of patient satisfaction [26,31-33], and significant improvement in preventative service utilization [26,31,33-35]. For example, Freeman *et al.* (1995) demonstrated that use of a patient navigator in an inner-city clinic yielded an 87.5% biopsy rate after an abnormal mammogram vs. a 56.6% biopsy rate in a clinic that did not use a patient navigator [26]. Frelix (1999) found similar results when a patient navigator in a low-cost screening center was used to coordinate return visits after an abnormal mammogram. In this study, the navigator enabled the program to show a detection rate of 12.9 per 1000 compared with the 5.1 per 1000 national detection rate [31]. Despite government initiatives and the onset of patient navigation programs within the health care setting, fundamental questions around the effectiveness, roles and responsibilities of a patient navigation program remain largely unanswered [29,30].

ONCOLOGY SOCIAL WORKERS AS PATIENT NAVIGATORS

The duties of the patient navigator are consistent with two core social work functions: empowering individuals to seek needed services and empowering communities to provide and improve those services [29]. Social workers have long navigated clients and communities toward improved social services, empowerment, and advocacy, making them an optimal choice in fulfilling the role of a patient navigator. Social workers have historically worked in communities to address social barriers that impede the well-being of underserved clients.

> "When I was first diagnosed, I didn't have any insurance and I didn't know where to turn. A lot of women don't know who to turn to for help. The first six months was really hard on me.... I wish someone could have helped me."

The social work profession is rooted in a social casework tradition adopted to address the inequality and fragmented nature of service delivery to the underserved [36,37]. Traditional case management is a collaborative process of assessment, planning, facilitation, and advocacy for options and services to meet an individual's health needs. Through communication and the procurement of available resources it promotes quality, cost-effective outcomes [38]. Patient navigation is grounded in the concepts of traditional case management. Oncology social workers need to embrace the concept of patient navigators and fight to claim this as the domain of social work. Oncology social workers have the professional values, training, and skills which make them naturally suited to assume a leading role in the patient navigation movement.

Chapter 3

STATE OF WOMENS' CANCERS

"My first thought when I was diagnosed with cancer was …Why me? … And, then I thought … Why not me? With this many women getting cancer, it's just the luck of the draw!"

WHY WOMENS' CANCERS?

Although each cancer type has its own unique impacts and complications, the main cancers classified as "women's cancers" have many similarities in the psychosocial impact on the lives of women. For this reason, each major type of women's cancers will be briefly reviewed for its impact on the lives of women, but then the psychosocial impact of these cancers will be reviewed collectively throughout the remainder of this book.

BREAST CANCER

Breast cancer continues to be the number one women's cancer in the United States and internationally. Breast cancer is the most common cancer in women, regardless of race or ethnicity [39]. In 2007, an estimated 178,480 women in the United States were diagnosed with breast cancer, and approximately 40,460 were expected to have died from breast cancer [40]. The incidence of breast cancer has increased from one in twenty in 1960 to one in eight today [40]. Fortunately, most women with breast cancer (almost 78%) survive the disease, primarily due to early diagnosis [41]. Breast cancer has been researched extensively, and researchers have found some important factors impacting the disease including: race/ethnicity, socioeconomic status, health factors, age, gender, and genetics.

OVARIAN CANCER

Ovarian cancer begins in the ovaries of the female reproductive system. Ovarian cancer is not the most common gynecologic malignancy, but it is the number one cause of deaths from gynecologic malignancy [41]. It is estimated that a woman's risk of getting invasive ovarian cancer during her lifetime is about 1 in 71 [42]. While the occurrence of ovarian cancer is relatively low, the mortality of the disease is not. Approximately 25,400 women in the U.S. are diagnosed with ovarian cancer each year, and each year approximately 14,300 women die from the disease [41]. Ovarian cancer is the eighth most common cancer among women, excluding non-melanoma skin cancers, and ovarian cancer accounts for about 3% of all cancers in women.

Ovarian cancer is the fifth leading cancer killer among women, accounting for more deaths than any other cancer of the female reproductive system. About three in four women with ovarian cancer survive at least one year after diagnosis, and almost half of the women with ovarian cancer are still alive at least five years after diagnosis. If ovarian cancer is diagnosed and treated before the cancer has spread outside the ovary, the 5-year survival rate is 92%. However, less than 20% of all ovarian cancers are found at this early stage [42]. Although ovarian cancer has not been studied as much as breast cancer, researchers have been able to find some important factors associated with the disease.

CERVICAL AND OTHER HPV CANCERS

Although cervical cancer is the most commonly diagnosed and widely known cancer caused by the human papilloma virus (HPV), other gynecological cancers are associated with HPV infection, including vaginal cancer and vulvar cancer. Each of these cancers is named for the site of primary malignancy: cervical cancer forms in the tissues of the cervix (the organ connecting the uterus and vagina); vaginal cancer forms in the vagina, or birth canal; and vulvar cancer forms in the tissues of the vulva (the external female genital organs) [43].

The American Cancer Society estimates that 11,070 new cases of cervical cancer will be diagnosed in 2008, resulting in 3,870 deaths. Between 1975 and 1992, the death rate from cervical cancer dropped by 74%, a decrease attributed to the introduction and increased use of the Pap screening test. This trend continues today, although less dramatically, as the death rate from cervical cancer decreases by almost 4% each year [43]. When detected and treated at its earliest stages, the present 5-year survival rate for cervical cancer is close to 92% [44]. Unfortunately, about half of all women in the U.S. do not receive regular Pap tests and screening for precancerous conditions, which may allow slow-growing and symptomless cervical cancer to develop undetected for many years [45]. As a result, the 5-year survival rate for all stages of cervical cancer combined is significantly lower, at about 72% [44].

Because they are diagnosed significantly less often than other women's cancer, less research has been dedicated to the study of vaginal and vulvar cancers. Vaginal cancer will account for approximately 2,210 new diagnoses and 760 deaths, while there will be close to 3,460 new cases and 870 deaths due to vulvar cancer [46]. Vaginal cancer makes up only 2% to 3% of all diagnoses of female reproductive cancers and, if detected in its earliest stages, can often be cured [44]. Vulvar cancer is only slightly more common, accounting for about 4% of female reproductive cancers and 0.6% of all cancers in women [46]. Although these cancers are less common and receive significantly less scientific and social attention than other female cancers, it is important to remember that they are taken no less seriously by a woman facing a diagnosis of vaginal or vulvar cancer. Accurate information about these cancers is scarce, even from authorities such as the American Cancer Society and the National Cancer Institute. Extra efforts should be made to connect women diagnosed with one of these cancers to appropriate information and resources, as they are unlikely able to find them on their own.

UTERINE CANCERS

Endometrial cancer is cancer that forms in the tissue lining of the uterus, while uterine sarcoma is a condition in which cancer cells form in the muscles of the uterus itself. Combined, these two uterine cancers are expected to account for 40,100 new cancer diagnoses and 7,470 deaths in 2008. Uterine sarcoma is much less common than endometrial cancer; more than 95% of diagnosed cancers of the uterus are endometrial cancer [47].

Endometrial cancer is the most common invasive cancer of the female reproductive system. A woman's total lifetime risk of developing endometrial cancer is 1 in 41. While incidence and mortality rates of endometrial cancer have remained relatively unchanged in recent years, statistics for uterine sarcoma have followed a somewhat different trend. Although there was a recorded increase in incidence rates of uterine sarcoma in the late 1980s to the late 1990s, these rates have been decreasing by approximately 1% per year since then. Additionally, while death rates saw an average decrease of 1.5% per year from 1975 to 1992, they have remained stable since that time [47].

Approximately 69% of uterine cancer cases are diagnosed while the cancer is still confined to the primary site. When detected at this early stage, the five-year survival rate for cancers of the uterus is 95.5%. The overall five-year survival rate for localized and metastasized uterine cancers is 82.9%. Racial disparities are evident in survival rates for this family of cancers: the five-year survival rate for Caucasian women is 84.7%, while black women have a significantly lower five-year survival expectation of 61.1% [48].

RISK FACTORS ASSOCIATED WITH WOMEN'S CANCERS

Race/Ethnicity

Racial and ethnic disparities are clear in all women's cancers. Breast cancer incidence and mortality rates vary greatly among different ethnic groups. In 2004, studies showed that Caucasian women had the highest incidence rate for breast cancer; African American women had the second highest incidence of getting breast cancer; followed by Asian/Pacific Islander, Hispanic, and American Indian/Alaska Native women [39]. Mortality rates from breast cancer indicate that African American women in the U.S. are more likely to die from breast cancer than any other racial/ethnic group [39].

One reason for the difference in mortality rate of African American women is due to the delay of seeking treatment. Studies suggest that African Americans are more likely to seek treatment only after a tumor has advanced, and that African American women generally do not avail themselves of early detection screening programs [49]. Other studies report similar screening behaviors among Hispanic women. This delay in screening and treatment results in breast cancer is the most common cause of death from cancer among Hispanic women [39].

Ovarian cancer incidence rates also vary among different ethnic groups. Statistics show that in 2004, Caucasian women had the highest incidence rate with about 14.3 per 100,000 women. Hispanic women are next highest with 11.5, followed by American Indian/Alaska Native with 11.2, African American women with 10.1, and lastly Asian/Pacific Islander with 9.7 in 100,000 women [50]. Furthermore, the death rate statistics for different ethnic groups in 2004 were as follows: Caucasian women with a rate of 9.2, African American women with 7.4, American Indian/Alaska Native with 7.1, Hispanic with 6.1, and Asian/ Pacific Islander with 4.8 per 100,000 women [50]. Statistics also show that five year survival rates are slightly higher for Caucasian women than African American women. African American women were also found to be significantly younger at the time of diagnosis and less likely to undergo site-specific surgery [51].

Significant racial and ethnic disparities are also evident in cervical cancer statistics. The rate of cervical cancer in the Hispanic population is more than twice that for non-Hispanic white women, and African American women are diagnosed with cervical cancer 50% more often than Caucasian women [43]. Even though Hispanic women have a significantly higher risk for developing cervical cancer, African American women are still at the greatest risk of dying of the disease. The death rate from cervical cancer for African American women is 4.7 per 100,000 women, compared with 3.2 for Hispanic women and 2.3 for non-Hispanic white women [44].

The risk of being diagnosed with, and dying of, vulvar cancer is greatest for non-Hispanic white women. The rate of diagnosis in this population is 2.3 per 100,000 women, compared with 1.9 for African American women and 1.7 for Hispanic women. The same trend holds true for mortality rates: non-Hispanic white women have the highest death rate at 0.5 per 100,000 women, while African American and Hispanic women have the same mortality rate of 0.3 per 100,000 women. Similar to trends documented in breast cancer literature, African American women are more likely to be diagnosed with endometrial cancer at a later stage of the disease's development. They are also more likely to die of this type of cancer than Caucasian women [48]. Caucasian and Asian women have similar rates of diagnosis of uterine sarcoma, but African American women are diagnosed about twice as often with this condition. Additionally, even when controlling for factors such as stage of diagnosis and course of treatment, African American women survive significantly fewer months and have a 26% greater chance of dying from uterine cancer when compared with white women. The reason for this disparity is not fully understood by researchers [47].

Race plays a key factor in medically uninsured rates with the rate for non-Hispanic Whites (10.8%) being significantly lower in 2006 compared to African Americans (20.5 %) and Hispanics (34.1% or 15.3 million) [52]. A recent study reported that race (white) and insurance status (private) are significant predictors of receiving a timely biopsy when presenting for cancer treatment. Findings imply that white women, with no history of previous breast cancer and private insurance are more likely to undergo aggressive evaluations than minority women with public or no insurance coverage [53,54].

Nationality

Cancer in women knows no borders and occurs worldwide. However, there are notable differences in the occurrence of these cancers around the world. For example, incidence rates of breast cancer are highest in industrialized nations such as the United States, Australia, and countries in Western Europe [55]. It is probable that global changes contribute to the differences of breast cancer occurrence in various countries. Also, the availability of medical treatment in less industrialized countries, as well as cultural differences, could contribute to the extreme differences in incidence rates reported. The lowest rates are found predominately in Asia and Africa, where the occurrence is less than twenty-five cases a year for every 100,000 women, as opposed to the United States and the Netherlands, which are five to eight times that amount [55]. While the rate of breast cancer appears dramatically different in Asia and Africa, it is difficult to get a true comparison of incidence numbers due to differences in diagnostic tools and tumor reporting among different countries [55].

One interesting study on migration reveals that when women from Japan move to the United States, their incidence of breast cancer increases six fold [49]. Even though this is a shocking increase, it is still lower than incidence rates for other women in the United States. This study has caused researchers to speculate that the switch from traditional Japanese dietary habits to the average American diet may be an important factor in explaining the dramatic difference [49].

Cervical cancer is a major health problem for women in developing countries. Of the 370,000 new cases of cervical cancer diagnosed each year, 80% to 85% are in developing countries, with the highest rates being found in Central America, South Asia, and sub-Saharan Africa. Cervical cancer accounts for 200,000 deaths in developing countries each year, making it the leading cause of cancer death among women in these countries. Much of this disparity can be traced to availability of screening and treatment for precancerous conditions. While 40% to 50% of women in developed countries receive regular Pap tests and screening for early signs of cervical cancer, it has been estimated that only about 5% of women in developing countries have received these same screening services. Experts predict that as life expectancies gradually increase for women in developing countries, there will be a corresponding increase in the number of diagnosed cervical cancer cases [45].

The differences that are found among ethnic groups appear to be related to cultural and environmental effects rather than genetic differences among ethnic groups [55]. There could be numerous reasons for differences in occurrence in ethnic groups. Some possible reasons of variation include: diet, socioeconomic status, and exposure to cancer causing agents. Some other differences in incidence and mortality rates of ethnic groups could be related to the time and stage of diagnosis. Varying cultural beliefs among ethnic groups may also be one cause of differences in medical treatment and diagnosis [55].

Socioeconomic Status

Socioeconomic status is another area that appears to impact cancer statistics. The role of socioeconomic status is complex and multifaceted. Poorer women are also less likely to have access to adequate health care providers and treatment, and are more likely to experience poor living conditions, poor diet, and less education. Socioeconomics may also play a large role in untested environmental risk factors that may be present in areas associated with high rates of poverty. Low-income women are less likely to utilize preventative screening programs (e.g., mammogram or Pap tests) to detect cancer in its earliest stage. Since the stage of cancer at diagnosis is the most important factor for survival, survival for low-income women is generally lower than other women from higher socioeconomic groups.

Poverty is a key factor driving health disparities [56-60]. Poverty is associated with a lack of resources and information, substandard living conditions, increased risk behaviors, and diminished access to health care [57]. In 2006, 36.5 million people were classified as living in poverty, and both the percentage and the number of people without health insurance increased in 2006 [52]. The percentage of individuals without health insurance increased from 15.3% in 2005 to 15.8% in 2006, and the number of medically uninsured increased from 44.8 million to 47.0 million. The medically underserved, regardless of insurance status, experience difficulties in accessing medical care throughout the continuum of cancer care. In 2000, Bickell and Chassin reported women enrolled in a Medicaid program and those having no insurance were at a higher risk of not receiving post breast-conserving surgery (BCS) radiation therapy and/or systematic chemotherapy. Findings also suggest uninsured women were less likely to receive radiation therapy after BCS and women insured by Medicaid were less likely to receive chemotherapy when compared to women with private insurance [61]. Health disparities are caused by a complex relationship between economic class, race/culture, and our current health care system [57,62].

Diet/Physical Activity

There are several health related topics including obesity, physical inactivity, diet, and alcohol use that impact incidence rates of cancer in women. Obesity has been found to be a risk factor for cancer in women. Studies have shown that overall, obese women have a higher risk of developing breast cancer, ovarian cancer, cervical cancer, and uterine cancer [39,43,63]. A nutritious diet is important for everyone's health, and may be helpful in the fight against women's cancers. Studies have shown conflicting results in the relationship of diet and women's cancer. For example, most studies have found that breast cancer is less common in countries where the typical diet is low in total fat, low in polyunsaturated fat, and low in saturated fat [63]. However, other studies have found no real correlation between fat intake and breast cancer. There is also research to suggest that women with diets low in fruits and vegetables and high in fats are at greater risk of developing cervical cancer and uterine cancer [43]. Although the research is limited, recent studies suggest that women who follow a low-fat diet for at least four years showed a lower risk of ovarian cancer [42]. Other studies show that women in the United States and Europe have a much higher incidence rate of ovarian cancer as opposed to women is other areas of the world, such as Japan [51]. These international statistics are believed to be due to the high-fat Western diet of animals, red meat, and dairy; however, more research is needed to confirm this claim. It is possible that the differences found in various countries could also be due to cultural and genetic differences.

Diabetes is considered a risk factor for cancer of the uterus, although the exact relationship between diabetes, weight, and cancer is still unknown. Diabetes is most often diagnosed in people who are overweight or obese, which could be why diabetic women are at a higher risk for developing endometrial cancer and uterine sarcoma. Some researchers, however, propose that diabetes itself could be a risk factor, regardless of a woman's weight [64].

Similarly, physical inactivity is believed to be a risk factor for cancer in women. Although there is currently little research on the relationship of physical exercise and cancer, the studies that have been done show that exercise can reduce the risk of breast cancer. Recent studies indicate that strenuous exercise in youth might provide lifelong protection against breast cancer, and that adults who engage in even moderate physical activity can lower their breast cancer risk [63].

While it is reported that alcohol consumption may be helpful in the fight against heart disease, it is shown to be quite the opposite when dealing with some of the cancers in women. For example, the use of alcohol is linked to an increased risk of developing breast cancer and higher consumption of alcoholic beverages results in higher breast cancer incidence [63,65]. Although it is not certain how alcohol may increase the risk for breast cancer, scientists believe that alcohol may influence the activity of hormones in the body, particularly estrogen [49,65]. As with many other types of cancer, smoking is also a risk factor for women's cancers. For example, smoking increases a woman's risk of developing cervical or other HPV-related cancers. Women who smoke are twice as likely as non-smokers to develop cervical cancer, and women infected with HPV greatly increase their risk of developing vaginal or vulvar cancer if they smoke [43].

Age

As women get older, their risk for cancer increases. Studies continue to show that aging remains one of the single greatest risk factors for the development of new cancers in women. The current median age for women diagnosed with breast cancer in the United States is 62 [55]. Older age also increases the risk of dying from breast cancer. Research shows that about 1 in 100 women who are 60 years old today will die from breast cancer by the age of 70 [39]. In 2005, roughly 11,110 women in the U.S. age 40 and under were projected to be diagnosed with breast cancer, and more than 1,400 of these were expected to die [66]. Although it has been shown that the incidence is lower in younger women compared to their older counterparts, the five-year survival rate is also lower due to tumors being more aggressive and less responsive to therapy [66]. Epidemiological studies suggest that younger women with breast cancer have worse disease-free and overall survival outcomes. At age 30, the probability of developing breast cancer in the next 10 years is 1 in 229. Currently there are more than 250,000 women in the United States under 40 living with breast cancer [66].

Like breast cancer, the risk of developing ovarian cancer increases with age. Studies from 2000-2004, showed that the median age at diagnosis of ovarian cancer was 63 years old, while 71 years old was the median age at death from ovarian cancer [50]. It is believed that women have an increased risk for ovarian cancer as they age due to changes in the cycle of ovulation and the process of menopause [51].

Cervical, vaginal, and vulvar cancers tend to be diagnosed in midlife. Most women with cervical cancer are diagnosed when they are younger than 50, with a median age of 48 at diagnosis [44]. Although cervical cancer is less common in women younger than 35, almost 20% of cervical cancer cases are diagnosed in women older than 65 [43]. More than two-thirds of women with vaginal cancer are 60 years old or older when diagnosed, with a median age of 69 at diagnosis [44]. Similarly, vulvar cancer tends to be diagnosed at midlife or later, with 85% of vulvar cancer cases diagnosed in women aged 50 or older. Half of all vulvar cancer cases are diagnosed in women over 70 [46].

Uterine cancers occur mainly in women over 50, with the largest percentage (28.8%) of cases diagnosed in women between the ages of 55 and 64. Less than 8% of these cancers are diagnosed in women under the age of 45, and 5.1% are diagnosed in women 85 years old or older. The median age of death from uterine cancers is 73 years of age, with the greatest percentage of deaths occurring between the ages of 75 and 84 [48].

Genetics

Family history is another important risk factor in most women's cancers. Genes can be inherited from both the mother and father and are passed along to both daughters and sons. The National Cancer Institute estimates that inherited gene mutations that are known to cause breast cancer account for only five to ten percent of the 211,000 cases that occur annually in the U.S. [49]. Women who inherit the mutated genes are generally diagnosed with breast cancer at a younger age, and are more likely to have aggressive tumors or have lost hormone receptors on the cells' surfaces, which in turn makes the disease more difficult to treat [49]. The two genes that are most known for causing breast cancer are BRCA1 and BRCA2. It is believed that about 50 to 60 percent of women with inherited BRCA1 or BRCA2 mutations will develop breast cancer by the age of 70 [63]. Since these genes are inherited from parents, men are also able to get the mutated genes. Studies show that about 20 percent of men diagnosed with breast cancer have a close male or female family member with breast cancer [55]. While male breast cancer only accounts for about 0.2 percent of all cancers in men [55], it is still important for men to be aware of the disease and its risk factors.

Family history of ovarian cancer is another high risk factor. A family history of ovarian cancer in a first-degree relative (a mother or a sister) or a second-degree relative (an aunt or a grandmother) makes a woman three to four times more likely to develop ovarian cancer. Studies show that the younger a relative is when she develops ovarian cancer, the higher the risk in future generations [42]. The risk also increases with the more relatives that have the disease. Research shows that about 10%-15% of ovarian cancers result from an inherited tendency to develop the disease. Furthermore, women who inherit genes with mutations also have an increased risk of developing breast cancer or colon cancer. Therefore, having a family member with breast cancer can also increase the risk of ovarian cancer [42].

Similarly, research suggests that a woman who has a first-degree relative (mother or sister) who has received a cervical cancer diagnosis in turn has a two to three times greater risk for developing the disease [43]. Doctors disagree, however, on the extent to which genetics play a role in this increased risk. Some researchers suggest that first-degree relatives are more likely to share some of the other environmental, lifestyle, or other non-genetic risk factors discussed in this section, which might have a more significant impact than DNA on a woman's risk of developing cervical cancer [67].

Although there does not appear to be a direct genetic link to endometrial cancer or uterine sarcoma risk, endometrial cancer seems to be more common in families who are frequently diagnosed with a certain type of colon cancer (hereditary nonpolyposis colorectal cancer, or HNPCC). Even though only a relatively small number of cases of endometrial cancer are associated with a history of colon cancer, genetic testing may be recommended for women who are identified as high risk due to a family history of colon cancer [68].

Reproductive History

Reproductive hormones are thought to impact cancer risk through effects on cell proliferation, DNA damage, and by promoting cancer growth [40]. Reproductive risk factors for breast and ovarian cancer include: early menstruation (before age 12), late menopause (after age 55), few or no pregnancies, and not breast feeding [40,41].

Oral contraceptives, tubal ligation and hysterectomy all have been found to decrease the risk of developing ovarian cancer. The repetitive ovulation theory proposed that the more times a woman ovulates during her lifetime, the more chances there are that a cell will undergo genetic damage that sets the cancer process in motion [51]. Studies have shown that taking oral contraceptives for five years can reduce ovarian cancer risk by as much as 50 percent. Researchers have found that progestin appears to play the key role in risk reduction. Some studies have found that it is possible that oral contraceptives continue to reduce the risk of developing ovarian cancer even years after women stop using them [51].

However, recent use of oral contraceptives may increase the risk of breast cancer, but the risk appears to decrease 10 years after a woman discontinues using oral contraceptives [40]. A woman increases her risk for developing cervical cancer by using oral contraceptives, and this risk continues to increase the longer she takes them. Research suggests, however, that the risk decreases after oral contraceptive use is stopped [43]. Since oral contraceptives have been shown to have both positive and negative impacts on a woman's risk of certain kinds of cancer, a woman should take this information into account when deciding whether to begin, continue, or stop oral contraceptive use.

Studies also have found that women who have either tubal ligation or hysterectomy procedures also have a small reduction in ovarian cancer risk. Despite widespread belief, researchers have reported that hysterectomies do not always eliminate the risk of ovarian cancer [51]. While these procedures may not fully eliminate the risk of ovarian cancer, it is important to remember that they do assist in reducing the risk.

Fertility drugs have also been hypothesized to increase the risk of ovarian cancer. Some studies have found that these drugs may increase ovarian cancer risk due to stimulating ovulation, especially when no pregnancy was able to occur [51]. Research suggests that fertility drugs increase the risk of low malignant ovarian tumors. However, other studies show no relationship between fertility drugs and ovarian cancer in infertile women; yet, researchers did find that infertility caused by unknown causes or endometriosis caused a higher risk of ovarian cancer [51]. It is evident that further studies need to be conducted to confirm if there is a relationship between fertility drugs and ovarian cancer.

Hormone replacement therapy (HRT) is also thought to increase a woman's cancer risk. New research has suggested that HRT, especially when used over long periods of time, may increase a woman's risk of developing breast and ovarian cancer [51]. Studies show that the risk increases when women use estrogens after menopause [42]. It is important that women discuss HRT with their physician before use.

Diethylstilbestrol (DES) was a commonly used hormonal drug between 1940 and 1971. Women during this time were given DES to prevent miscarriage and reduce pregnancy and delivery complications. The next generation of women, whose mothers were given DES while pregnant, have a higher incidence of reproductive cancers than is seen in the general population. DES exposure appears to have a stronger association with vaginal than cervical cancer, although more than 40% of women diagnosed with vaginal cancer have no history of in utero DES exposure. This is a relatively minor risk factor, as less than 1% of women exposed to DES have developed a reproductive cancer. Additionally, as many of these women have gotten older and passed the age of highest risk for cervical cancer, researchers predict a decline in the number of women's cancer cases attributed to DES exposure.

Unlike breast and uterine cancers, where pregnancy lowers a woman's risk of developing cancer, multiple full-term pregnancies increases a woman's risk for cervical cancer [43]. Although research has not offered conclusive evidence for this association, several theories have been suggested. For example, some researchers believe that these women have had more exposure to HPV strains through more frequent sexual contact. Other experts believe that the hormonal changes that occur in a woman's body during pregnancy temporarily weaken her immune system, making her more susceptible to HPV infection during that time [43].

A woman's reproductive history also influences her risk of developing endometrial cancer and uterine sarcoma. Starting menstrual periods before the age of 12, never becoming pregnant or never giving birth, or going through natural menopause later in life all increase a woman's risk of developing a cancer of the uterus [47]. Under these conditions, a woman's body is exposed to estrogen for a longer, uninterrupted amount of time, and cancers of the uterus are predominantly estrogen-driven [69].

At one time, estrogen was prescribed to menopausal woman to treat the common symptoms of hot flashes and thinning bones, and to replace the estrogen no longer produced by the ovaries. Doctors now recognize that this type of hormone replacement therapy (HRT) increases a woman's risk of developing several cancers, including endometrial cancer [48]. To counteract this unintended consequence, post-menopausal women are commonly prescribed estrogen-progestin replacement therapy, in which estrogen is combined with progesterone, another naturally occurring hormone. While this reduces the therapy's impact on endometrial cancer risk, adding progesterone to estrogen-only HRT actually increases a woman's risk for developing breast cancer and blood clots [47]. Taking oral contraceptives that combine estrogen and progestin similarly impact the risk of developing endometrial cancer and breast cancer respectively. The protective effect of these combination oral contraceptives has been shown to last for many years, even after a woman stops using them [48].

HUMAN PAPILLOMA VIRUS (HPV)

HPV is associated with the majority of cases of cervical, vaginal, and vulvar cancers. There are more than 100 different strains of HPV and about 30 of these have been shown to cause these gynecological cancers [70]. Two particular strains (HPV 16 and PHV 18) are thought to be responsible for more than two-thirds of new cervical cancer cases [43]. While HPV infection is the most significant risk factor for cervical cancer, only a small percentage of women infected with HPV will develop the disease [44]. Vaginal cancer has been associated with the same types of HPV that cause cervical cancer, with between 65% and

80% of vaginal cancers caused by the HPV virus [46]. In the case of vulvar cancer, however, research suggests that there might be two distinct types of the disease. Many cases of vulvar cancer in younger women can be attributed to HPV infection, but this is less of a concern in elderly women diagnosed with the disease. Studies suggest that the vulvar cancer diagnosed in older women has no association with the HPV virus [46].

Promising advances have been made in the development of vaccines to prevent HPV infection. Several vaccines are in varying stages of development but, for now, only one has received approval by the U.S. Food and Drug Administration. This vaccine, Gardasil, protects against four types of HPV that are thought to cause two-thirds of all cervical cancers. Although the vaccine is being marketed for its ability to lower cervical cancer risk, it also has potential benefits for vaginal and vulvar cancers that share a common HPV source [71].

Women with a history of sexually transmitted diseases, such as chlamydia, gonorrhea, or syphilis, are at higher risk of developing cervical cancer. It is thought that women who have acquired sexually transmitted diseases have had a greater number of sexual partners or engaged in unsafe sex practices, thereby putting themselves at greater risk for HPV infection [72]. Women with weakened immune systems appear to be at greater risk for cervical and other HPV-related cancers [72]. This includes women who are positive for the human immunodeficiency virus (HIV), the virus that causes AIDS. HIV damages the body's immune system, making it more vulnerable to infections, including HPV infection [43].

MULTIPLE CANCERS

Having one type of cancer can be a risk factor for developing another type of cancer. Cervical, vaginal, and vulvar cancers have numerous similar risk factors, most notably HPV infection. A diagnosis of one of these cancers increases the likelihood that a woman will be diagnosed with another HPV-related cancer based on these common risk factors [43]. Although the exact relationship is still unclear, women who have been diagnosed with breast or ovarian cancer appear to have a higher risk of developing endometrial cancer as well [47]. In addition, certain ovarian diseases develop estrogen-producing tumors, which results in elevated levels of estrogen and lower than normal levels of progesterone. As discussed in a previous section, this increased exposure to estrogen in the body raises a woman's risk for developing endometrial cancer and uterine sarcoma [47].

One possible association between ovarian conditions and endometrial cancer is the use of pelvic radiation therapy to treat the primary ovarian disease. The use of high-energy radiation, particularly in the pelvic area, can damage the DNA of healthy cells, increasing a woman's risk of developing a second kind of cancer [47]. These secondary cancers have been documented anywhere from five to 25 years after initial exposure to the radiation, so long-term monitoring is recommended for women who have received this type of therapy [48].

Tamoxifen, a drug often used in the treatment of women with breast cancer or to reduce the risk of developing the disease in women who have been identified as high-risk, behaves like estrogen in the uterus by causing the uterine lining to grow [47]. Use of this therapy, therefore, increases a woman's risk of developing a cancer of the uterus. Approximately 1 in 500 women who take tamoxifen will develop endometrial cancer, so this relatively small risk should be weighed against the advantages of its uses in treating or reducing the risk of developing breast cancer [73].

CONCLUSIONS

The risks factors associated with women's cancer are often confusing for survivors and their families. Women often question why this happened to them or wonder what they did wrong. They might also be concerned about the risks for their daughters, sisters, and other loved ones. It is important for oncology social workers to understand the risk factors associated with these cancers and connect survivors and their families to appropriate resources to help them understand their disease.

> "I just can't understand why I got this disease …. I am a vegetarian, I exercise, and I breast fed my babies! I tried to do everything right. It just isn't fair."

A referral to genetic counseling may also be appropriate for some women and families. By identifying risks for the disease and detecting cancers early, genetic counseling and testing can dramatically improve the chances of surviving breast cancer. However, deciding to undergo genetic testing is a very personal and complex matter which needs to be given careful consideration.

> "Everybody in my family has breast cancer – my sister, my mom, my grandma. I hope my daughter doesn't get it too. The doctor wanted us to do the genetic counseling, but my daughter said that she just didn't want to know. She said that she is just going to leave it in God's hands."

Genetic counseling and testing is often not covered by insurance, so there may be a considerable financial cost for women. In addition, women and their families are often concerned about the impact that genetic testing may have on their ability to get health insurance, disability insurance, and life insurance. The oncology social worker can be beneficial in discussing these issues with women and their loved ones and making appropriate referrals to genetic counselors.

Chapter 4

DIFFERENT FACES OF CANCER

"Someone said to me 'You don't look like a cancer patient'. And I said, 'Well, what does a cancer patient look like?'

YOUNGER WOMEN WITH CANCER

As the incidence of cancer in young women is generally much lower than in older women, it has been shown that young women are an underrepresented population in many research studies. Despite widespread opinion, cancer in young women can and does occur, thus the need for more research on this underserved population is crucial [40].

In addition to the physical suffering experienced by women diagnosed with cancer, there is considerable emotional suffering for these women and their families. A woman with cancer is likely to be faced with multiple concerns during her diagnosis and treatment of cancer such as, coping with treatments, financial strain, childcare issues, employment concerns, and future health concerns. Although cancer can be stressful for all women, younger women are likely to face unique concerns and may be particularly in need of additional support [74,75]. For younger women and single women, perceived social support has been positively associated with quality of life and adjustment to cancer [76,77].

"I had lumps in my breast and begged for a mammogram for years, but the doctors kept telling me I was too young for breast cancer and too young to have a mammogram. When they finally listened to me, I was in the last stages and now I'm going to die."

It has also been shown that younger women with cancer have a higher risk for significant psychological distress, including mood disturbance, anxiety, depression, and other psychosocial symptoms requiring intervention [78-81]. Younger women appear more vulnerable to greater disruption to their daily lives and have greater unmet practical needs, such as child care. These women struggle with many issues that their post-menopausal counterparts do not face, such as the possibility of early menopause, difficulty of pregnancy after diagnosis, higher mortality rates, and more aggressive tumors.

"At the age of 42, I thought ... Am I going to get a husband? I can see somebody sticking with me after we've been married and this happens, but now ...?

In addition to the distress a cancer diagnosis and subsequent treatments bring with it, younger women are more likely to be simultaneously engaged in multiple life roles that their older counterparts may have left behind. These roles include starting a family, caring for dependent children, being a student, working full- or part-time outside of the home, and being a wife/domestic partner/girlfriend. Juggling these responsibilities presents a challenge for any young woman. When a woman receives a cancer diagnosis, not only must she come to grips with her disease, she must also cope with how such a diagnosis will disrupt the many roles in which she is engaged. For many women, the thought of not surviving to see their children grow up is an overwhelming concern that brings with it great sadness [78,82].

"All I could think about when I was diagnosed with advanced cancer was that I'm not going to live to raise my children. It is an overwhelming thought."

Women who are not currently mothers but who hope to become so at some point face their own set of concerns in light of a cancer diagnosis. While cancer itself may not affect fertility, the adjuvant therapies (including radiation therapy and chemotherapy) used to treat it can potentially do so. Younger women with cancer may experience treatments that bring about not only premature menopause, but also the onset of vaginal dryness, mood swings, hot flashes, and short term memory loss [79]. Young women with cancer cite potential infertility as being a major concern for them [82,83]. A woman's conception of what is feminine and young often includes the ability to bear children, should they make the choice to do so. To have this ability taken away from them as result of the treatment for their cancer can be devastating.

"I was young and just dating. If I have a mastectomy, who it going to accept me? Once you're married, you expect sickness and health, but not when you are dating."

It is important that women who think they may want to have children after they are finished with their cancer treatments talk to their doctors about their options. Previously, doctors tended to suggest that survivors should not attempt to get pregnant after they are cancer-free because it was thought that the increased levels of estrogen and progesterone present in a woman's body when she is pregnant would encourage cancer re-growth. However multiple studies have shown that post-cancer pregnancy has no effect on the mother's survival [84-86]. If a woman still has her period after cancer treatment has ended, she may still be able to have children [87]. Younger women should be encouraged to discuss their plans and options for having children with their treatment team prior to undergoing cancer treatment.

"God, if I have another baby it is going to come out with six ears after all the toxic stuff I've had in my body. I'm really afraid!"

A loss of fertility is not the only way in which a woman who has been diagnosed with cancer might find her notions of femininity challenged. For example, for many women breasts are central to their sense of femininity. Her body image and sense of femininity may suffer a significant blow if she undergoes a mastectomy, in which one or both breasts are surgically removed. Breast conserving surgery (lumpectomy), in which a tumor or tumors are cut out of the breast tissue while leaving healthy breast tissue intact, may leave breasts looking significantly changed post-surgery, especially if a large amount of cancerous tissue is removed. Women report feeling "disfigured" and "not like a woman" after such procedures [79]. Options for breast reconstruction should be discussed with all women at the time of diagnosis and throughout the treatment process. At the time of diagnosis, women are often focused on just surviving the cancer, but after treatment is completed, they may once again begin to focus on fertility issues and breast reconstruction. Therefore, it is important for oncology social workers and the treatment team to revisit these issues with women throughout the continuum of care.

African American Women with Cancer

African American women suffer a disproportionate burden from women's cancer. African American women have higher mortality rates compared to Caucasian women for most women's cancers [88]. African American women are also more likely to be diagnosed with advanced stages of cancer and at a younger age [40,88-90]. The five year survival rates are significantly poorer for African American women compared to Caucasian women for most women's cancers [40]. Poorer survival can be attributed to both late stage diagnosis and poorer stage-specific survival [40]. According to several review studies [30,62], there are numerous factors that contribute to these health disparities, such as lack of health insurance [91-98] or regular source of care [99,100], low levels of health literacy [96,98,101,102], cultural beliefs [98,99,103-106], and logistic barriers (e.g., transportation, childcare, work schedule) [93,98,102,104,107,108].

The differences in incidence of and mortality from cancer in Caucasian and African American women have been attributed, at least in part, to the lower rate of preventative screening among African American women. For example, several studies have been conducted comparing African American women who did and who did not regularly obtain a mammogram [101,102,109-111]. Husaini and colleagues (2001) found that age, marriage, educational intervention, talking with friends, and accurate knowledge about breast cancer all had a positive impact on African American women obtaining a mammogram, while depression had a negative impact. Crump and colleagues (2000) found that age, attitudinal factors, and referral source were key factors predicting whether African American women obtained a mammogram. In addition, Davis and colleagues found that not being instructed by a doctor to get a mammogram was the primary reason that low-income African American women had not obtained a mammogram on a yearly basis [102].

> "I went to the doctors, but they never told me to get a mammogram. My mom didn't have breast cancer and my grandma didn't have breast cancer. No one in my family had cancer. I didn't think I needed to get my breast checked and then I found a lump."

Oncology social workers can play a key role in facilitating programs to target preventative screenings for African American women. For example, an oncology social worker developed an African American specific outreach program titled "Hats Off to Breast Cancer" which uses culturally sensitive skits to teach African American women about cancer risks. These skits are performed in African American churches and community centers in low-income urban areas [112].

Hispanic Women with Cancer

Similar to African American women, the state of cancer for Hispanic women is bleak. Breast cancer is the primary cause of cancer deaths among Hispanic women despite their having overall lower incidence rates of the disease compared to non-Hispanic White and African American women [113]. Hispanic women have also been found to be diagnosed at more advanced stages of breast and cervical cancer compared to other population groups [114]. In fact, a 2003 study revealed that Hispanic whites, African Americans and American Indians had 1.7- to 2.5-fold elevations in risk of stage III and stage IV tumors in comparison to non-Hispanic whites [115]. Since survival rates are directly linked to the diagnosis stage, the five-year survival rate for Hispanic women with cancer in contrast to non-Hispanic white women is significantly poorer [114,116]. These statistics are indicative of documented low early detection screening participation rates and inadequate medical care [116-119].

A number of factors have been pinpointed as contributing to the underutilization of cancer preventive and palliative care resources by Hispanic women. Leading among them are poverty, lack of quality health care, and misunderstandings about cancer from an educational and cultural perspective [117,119-122]. Hispanics will fill nearly a quarter of the Nation's population by the year 2050 [118,123], yet there is a disproportionate amount of research on the impact of cancer and quality of life for Hispanic women [118].

Hispanics represent around 12% of the population but they make up 25% of America's uninsured. The 1999 unemployment rate for Hispanics was 6.7%, compared to 3.6% for non-Hispanic Whites [123]. It has been reported that Hispanics utilize emergency room treatment more frequently because they are almost three times less likely to have a consistent source of medical care. In fact, compared to the general population, Hispanics are 1.5 times more likely to rely on the hospital emergency room as their primary source of care. In addition, uninsured Hispanics are two to three times more likely to have cancer diagnosed at a more advanced stage, rendering it less treatable. Hispanic women who are uninsured are reported to be 2.3 times more likely to be diagnosed with breast cancer at a later stage. Minimal access to care and comparatively unsatisfactory medical outcomes are obvious health risks threatening uninsured Hispanics. Uninsured Hispanics are less likely to have a regular source of medical care, less likely to have regular visits to a physician, and less likely to use preventive services. Subsequently, they are more likely to delay seeking medical care and to report having not received necessary care [124].

> "As a social worker, I took one of my Hispanic patients to all of her radiation/chemotherapy appointments as well as to her surgery for her mastectomy and she never told her family and would not allow the doctors to tell anyone. She was so ashamed."

In congruence with the findings on uninsured Hispanics, slightly more than half (52.6 %) of Hispanic women age 40 and older have had regular mammogram screenings in the past year [114]. A 2006 study exploring the breast cancer knowledge and beliefs of Hispanics living in Houston, Texas revealed that more than a third of the 63 participants viewed breast cancer as fatal, 29% believed pain signalized onset of the disease and 11.1% had never heard of breast cancer [125].

> "When I was diagnosed the first thing that came to my mind and stayed in my mind was that I would die. I kept thinking of never seeing my grandkids again."

Other documented cancer-related misperceptions of Hispanic women include the idea that bumps, bruises and surgery cause cancer [126]. Such inaccuracies have a direct effect on preventive health behaviors [126]. Language barriers are also continually cited as influencing Hispanic women's underutilization of screening services [118,125]. Women who are capable of speaking English and who opt to speak English instead of Spanish have a higher chance of receiving a mammogram [118]. Research has also demonstrated how attitudes and beliefs specific to the Hispanic culture also influenced the potential impact of cancer. Modesty, emphasis on privacy concerning ailments, and assumptions that cancer is contagious or a life sentence from God were cited as contributing to low cancer screenings for Hispanic women. Findings also revealed that Hispanics' consciousness of cancer is raised through close friends and family friends who are educated on cancer issues [118].

> "In this country people are more open to know everything, but in my country it is like a secret. It is like discrimination, like when someone has AIDS ... they hide it."

In order to decrease the disparities of cancer for Hispanic women, culturally sensitive educational outreach strategies are needed in Hispanic communities [118,125-127]. Oncology social workers are in a key position to advocate for services to meet the needs of Hispanic cancer survivors and their families.

> "I would like someone who is willing to help in the most difficult moments, who will support me, who will understand my language when I go to the clinic. Everything is in English and I don't understand what they are saying. I need someone who speaks my language that can help me."

Other Populations

Ethnic and minority women face unique obstacles in receiving appropriate screening and treatment for cancer. The research literature on cancer in minority populations focuses primarily on Hispanic or African American women, ignoring several other ethnic minority groups of considerable size, such as Asian Americans (including Koreans, Vietnamese, Filipinos, and Indians), Native Hawaiians and Pacific Islanders, American Indians, and Alaska Natives. The scarcity of research related to these other minority groups is frustrating not only to the women of these groups searching for culturally sensitive and appropriate information for their cancer diagnosis, but also to the professionals who question how to provide meaningful services to these clients.

Although women's cancers are a significant health concern among ethnic and minority populations, women in these groups tend to view cancer as a "white woman's disease," making it less likely that they will seek regular screening and timely follow-up [128]. The stigma associated with this mindset is present in both the women diagnosed with the cancers and those in their larger communities, potentially influencing the course of treatment as women worry about how their diagnosis will be received by family and friends. Many women from minority ethnic communities report that cancer is a taboo subject and therefore not openly discussed within a community. For a woman diagnosed with cancer, this stigma results in isolation that can lead to feelings of depression and uncertainty [129]. This sense of "other" is further perpetuated by interactions with doctors and other medical staff, who often treat minority women in a paternalistic way, overlook the consequences of significant language barriers, or rush patients into making medical decisions based on principles of Western medicine rather than traditional methods with which the woman might be more familiar [128].

> "In my culture, we don't discuss things like breast cancer openly like in this country. I didn't even want to tell my family when I was diagnosed with cancer. I felt very ashamed and did not want to disappoint my family."

Several risk factors associated with different forms of cancer are especially prevalent in minority female populations, including lower levels of education, greater levels of poverty, and reduced access to regular screening and early detection [130].While diet and lifestyle practices in their home country might have served as protective factors, acculturation into mainstream Western society has been shown to rapidly increase a woman's risk for developing cancer [130-132]. The changes to diets high in animal fat and reduced physical activity have the greatest impact on increased cancer risk. While many minority women transition into more Western diet and exercise routines, many women also retain customs and beliefs from their country of origin in regards to health care practices. They may delay or avoid screening and treatment for a number of reasons (including religious beliefs or accessibility), or turn to traditional healing methods (such as herbal therapy) in times of illness [131,133]. In other words, while an ethnic minority woman may become acculturated into a Western diet and lifestyle, adopting Western beliefs about health and healing comes far more slowly, putting these women in a dangerous place in terms of developing and detecting cancer.

Native Hawaiians and Pacific Islanders

Although Pacific Islanders comprise a small portion of the total U.S. population (0.1%), there is still a great deal of diversity in this group which includes Native Hawaiians, Samoans, Chamorros, Tongans, Fijians, and other smaller groups [134]. Overall cancer rates within the Pacific Islanders population are generally lower than rates for non-Hispanic whites, but cancer, particularly of the breast and cervix, tends to be diagnosed at a later stage, which results in increased mortality [135]. Native Hawaiian women fare worst among all Pacific Islander groups in both incidence and mortality rates: they have the highest incidence and mortality of endometrial cancer, the third highest breast cancer mortality rate, and a significantly higher uterine cancer mortality rate despite lower overall incidence of uterine cancer [134]. The overall cancer death rate for Native Hawaiian and Samoan women exceeds that of non-Hispanic White women, with the greatest number of deaths attributed to breast cancer [135].

American Indians and Alaska Natives

As with Pacific Islanders, there is great diversity within the American Indian and Alaska Native population, which is made up of more than 560 federally recognized tribes and over 100 state recognized tribes [136]. Although American Indian and Alaska Native groups historically have had lower cancer rates than the general U.S. population, there has been a steady increase in cancer rates for these groups in the past 20 years. Part of this increase may be explained by previous misclassification of American Indians and Alaska Natives as either White or Hispanic in data collection and literature. While official forms now offer a category for American Indians and Alaska Natives to classify themselves, traditional methods of documentation did not allow for these distinctions, causing many members of these groups to classify themselves in a category that did not match their tribal identification. Another difficulty arises when members of these populations must identify themselves as a generic group labeled "other." This label encompasses numerous groups that do not identify as White, African American, or Hispanic, which makes tracking and detecting changes in cancer rates impossible. Some studies suggest that there is as much as 40-50% official misclassification of members of these groups [136].

Regardless of the effect of classification on cancer rates, there is no doubt that cancer is a growing health concern for members of these groups. Alaska Natives have one of the highest combined cancer mortality rates when compared with other racial groups, and both groups have the poorest cancer survival rates. While rates of breast cancer for these groups are comparable to the general U.S. population, women in these groups have disproportionately higher rates of less common women's cancers. For example, rates of cervical cancer are unusually high for both Alaska Native women and Northern Plains American Indians. Until culturally-targeted educational programs reach women of these populations, it is likely that these cancer rates will continue to increase.

Asian Americans

Cancer has been the leading cause of death for Asian American women since 1980. Asian American women were the first American population to have this unfortunate distinction, despite the fact that rates of breast and other cancers in their countries of origin are the lowest in the world [137]. As previously discussed, changes in diet and lifestyle are predominantly responsible for the dramatic increase in cancer rates among this diverse population. In fact, as a result of these changes, breast cancer incidence in Japanese American women is quickly approaching that of White women. Breast cancer is among the top three most frequently diagnosed cancers in subgroups of Asian American women [135].

While breast cancer is a significant health problem for all groups of Asian American women, cervical cancer is also quite common among these groups. Both incidence and mortality due to cervical cancer have increased for Asian American women in the past 10 years [138]. Southeast Asian women have higher rates of cervical cancer (as well as lower screening frequency) than almost all other U.S. ethnic groups [137]. Cervical cancer is among the most diagnosed cancers in Korean, Laotian, and Kampuchean women, and the most frequently diagnosed cancer in Vietnamese women living in the U.S., at a rate five times higher than non-Hispanic White women [135,137]. As seen in other ethnic minority cultures, an Asian American woman's role within her family often takes precedence over her health care needs, leading her to neglect regular screening practices for cervical cancer. Also present in other cultures is the belief that discussing sexual practices is taboo and that receiving cervical cancer screening implies inappropriate sexual activity [138]. These beliefs have far-reaching impacts on the health of Asian American women, as evidenced in increasing rates of cervical cancer within this group.

> "We do not feel comfortable talking about our bodies in our culture like Western women here. The women in my family do not go for female exams because they are embarrassed."

In terms of interactions with their health care team, Asian American women tend to prefer taking a passive role. Many Asian American women defer treatments about their course of cancer treatment to their physician. This is especially true of monolingual women, who face particular barriers in communicating with their care team and receiving the information they need to make an informed decision. Interestingly, in at least one study, Asian American women expressed greater satisfaction with their interactions with their doctor than did White, Hispanic, or African American women [138]. While many Asian American women may seem comfortable handing over their treatment decisions, this deference should not be assumed. In fact, more acculturated Asian American women feel that women should play a more active role in information-seeking and decision-making when it comes to their health care. It is important, therefore, for the oncology social worker to work with the Asian American client to be sure that she understands her rights in the decision-making and treatment process.

Additionally, some Asian American groups prefer gentler, indirect forms of communication, such as eye contact and smiling. In one study of Filipino cancer patients, participants reported their discomfort at the directness of everyone in the medical setting, from the physician to the hospital priest. Even though they recognized that the information was truthful and necessary, they were disappointed to not receive any sympathy or recognition of their personal struggle with their situation [139]. The Filipino women also said that they tend to hide their feelings about their cancer diagnosis; they come from a country where life is difficult for most people, which developed in them a certain degree of toughness in facing life's struggles. But while they may be able to put their diagnosis in perspective to those around them, it is nonetheless important for the oncology social worker (and other members of the health care team) to take a moment to check on their emotional state, regardless of how strong they may appear. As one Filipino cancer patient said, "Sometimes it helps just to ask, 'How are you doing?'" [139].

Rural Women with Cancer

Although the medical and social science literature contains literally thousands of studies exploring the physical and psychosocial impact of a cancer diagnosis on women, the vast majority of those studies were conducted with urban women in urban treatment centers [140]. This ignores the different demands that a cancer diagnosis has for women living in rural regions, often with limited medical and support resources.

"I was given some information about support groups, but I wasn't going to drive all that way just to go to some group. I could barely make it for my treatments. There was none of that stuff in my area."

Rural women face disproportionately higher rates of cancer diagnoses when compared with national averages. For example, the rates of women's cancers are significantly higher in parts of Appalachia than the rest of the country. Central Appalachia has a cervical cancer rate 35% higher than the rest of the country, while the rate of uterine cancer in northern Appalachia is 34% higher, and ovarian cancer is 12% higher for the region as a whole [141]. Despite the high rates for cervical, uterine and ovarian cancers, invasive breast cancer is still the most commonly diagnosed malignancy for women in Appalachia. In addition, women in this region have significantly higher death rates from cervical cancer and for all cancer sites combined.

Some of this disparity can be linked to screening behaviors. Women with lower incomes tend to delay preventive screenings, either for economic reasons or for lack of easily accessible screening facilities. Similarly, older women and women with lower education in Appalachia are less likely to participate in regular Pap tests and mammography screenings [141]. This lack of screening translates into more advanced cancers at time of diagnosis and higher death rates.

Also contributing to cancer disparities in rural women is the fact that rural populations tend to have higher rates of poverty than the general population. Previous studies have indicated that cervical cancer is associated with high rates of poverty such as that found in Appalachia [141]. In addition to presenting a barrier to accessing screening services, poverty can affect treatment options, mental health, and quality of life for rural women diagnosed with cancer [142]. Rural, low-income women tend to hold jobs requiring less education and fewer job-specific skills, which makes missing long periods of work to travel for cancer treatment a significant concern. The stress of uncertain employment status, added to the emotional strain of a cancer diagnosis, has been linked with higher levels of depression and lower self-reported quality of life. Furthermore, rural, low-income survivors with cancer are less likely to receive mental health services, such as treatment for depression and prescription of antidepressant medications [142].

In a literature review of the limited studies of the needs of rural cancer patients and survivors, findings revealed that the course of cancer treatment for women living in rural areas often differs markedly from that of urban women, even when tumor size and stage of diagnosis are comparable [140]. For example, studies show that rural women with a breast cancer diagnosis are significantly more likely to receive mastectomy and chemotherapy, and less likely to undergo lumpectomy and receive radiation therapy, when compared with urban women. Similarly, rural woman are less likely to receive adjuvant therapy as often as National Cancer Institute standards recommend [143]. Studies suggest that physicians have a strong influence on the treatment decisions of female cancer patients, as women often defer choices about the course of treatment to the physician's professional opinion. This may be particularly true for rural cancer patients, who report having less access to relevant cancer-related information, including treatment options and the stage of their own cancer [144].

"I told the doctor just to take my breast off. I couldn't afford to come in everyday for treatments. I just wanted to get it over with and get back to normal."

This lack of information is present not only for rural cancer patients, but also for rural physicians as well. The main reason that rural cancer patients must travel to urban treatment facilities is that appropriate facilities are not available locally. Upon completing primary treatment and returning to the care of their local physicians, many women find that their physicians lack up-to-date knowledge about oncology-related issues [145,146]. Rural physicians may choose to consult with urban cancer specialists who remotely treat rural cancer survivors; however, the quality of communication varies greatly. If the communication is poor, the rural cancer survivor is more likely to report a lack of adequate medical care [144].

Travel is a significant factor in the rural cancer survivor's treatment. For example, one focus group study of rural breast cancer survivors revealed that half of the participants had traveled one hour for surgery, while one-quarter had traveled more than three hours. In this same sample, a significant number reported traveling more than three hours for chemotherapy (21%) and radiation (61%) [144]. While the distance between a rural cancer survivor's home and an urban treatment center may impact treatment choices (as previously discussed), rural women who are able to receive appropriate care locally feel more positive about their provider and their overall experience than those who must travel farther away to receive care [147]. Not surprisingly, traveling long distances for surgery, chemotherapy, or radiation adds to the stress and exhaustion of the cancer diagnosis and treatment. Rural cancer survivors often find themselves in unfamiliar large cities, having been given little practical advice on how to travel to or within the city, or how to locate affordable accommodation near the treatment facility [140,148].

> "The worst part was driving so far to get the treatments. It was an entire day and sometimes I had to stay overnight. It was hard for me and my whole family. I was so far away from my doctors."

One benefit for rural cancer survivors who travel to urban treatment centers is the opportunity to interact with other cancer survivors. Rural breast cancer patients, for example, have reported numerous advantages to these interactions, including minimizing fears, reducing feelings of isolation, and developing a positive survivorship perspective [147,149]. Unfortunately, after developing supportive relationships with other cancer survivors in urban treatment centers, many rural women report a significant loss of social support when they return home. In their own rural communities, women report feeling isolated and stigmatized as a result of their cancer diagnosis. These feelings are increased amid concerns about privacy and gossip about their health status [150-152]. Further contributing to this social strain is limited availability of formal mental health services, which are often inaccessible for financial or geographic reasons. Even when mental health services are available, the stigma associated with utilizing them prevents many women from receiving the support they need to adjust to life during and after cancer treatment [144].

In addition to issues of social support, rural cancer survivors must also contend with practical concerns of daily life. Being absent for days or weeks at a time to receive cancer treatment causes noticeable disruptions in employment and family life. While juggling the obligations of running a household and caring for children can be difficult for any woman facing a cancer diagnosis, it is especially so for women living in rural communities, where assistive services (such as formal childcare or house-cleaning services) are less available

[144,148]. Rural cancer survivors frequently report difficulties fulfilling their gender-specific roles and are concerned about becoming a burden, rather than a caretaker, to their family. At the same time, however, many of these women say they would like additional support from family members [153]. Oncology social workers should take care to avoid the assumption that all small communities join together to help a family member or neighbor in need, and instead explore all avenues of social and practical support available to the rural cancer survivor. Given that rural survivors are unlikely to have an oncology social worker or any social worker available locally, it might be useful to provide telephone counseling to these women throughout the continuum of care.

Advanced Stage Cancer and Recurrence of Cancer

Advanced stage cancer or a recurrence is often the most difficult news to discuss with the survivor and her family. Making decisions on cancer treatment is especially difficult because several treatment modalities exist, each with associated risks and benefits. The decision making process is highly stressful as patients are asked to consider an enormous amount of information, learn a new language, and make life changing decisions. The emotional and physical impact on the survivor when prognosis is poor is often overwhelming. Oncology social workers are particularly important during this phase of care.

> "I didn't know I had any emotions –they flattened when I found out the cancer returned. I couldn't do any of that (make decisions, communicate). I was just finished."

Although the survivor literature tends to discuss advanced and recurring cancer simultaneously, a diagnosis of cancer recurrence carries its own unique set of issues with which survivors and their families must cope. While survivors with advanced cancer must face practical and emotional end-of-life decisions, those with a cancer recurrence must face the sometimes equally overwhelming idea of resumed treatments and the possibility of never "getting better." Researchers and doctors agree that, in many cases, cancer can now be treated as a chronic condition rather than something that must be aggressively cured. This is welcome news to some cancer survivors, who are comforted by the idea of a longer life expectancy even if it means continued treatments to manage the disease and its symptoms. Other survivors, however, are physically and emotionally exhausted from their previous cancer battles and question if they have the strength to endure the entire process again [154].

> "You're flat lined when it hits you again. I'm terrified now. I'm going to die. It is much harder the second time around."

For some cancer survivors, the fear of recurrence is emotionally stressful in the long-term survivorship phase. Many women report feeling abandoned when treatment ends and they are only required to have annual check-ups with their oncologist [155]. Although they may not recognize it until after treatment ends, women often feel a sense of comfort in seeing their oncologist regularly during the course of treatment, confident that the doctor will detect any stray cancer cells in their earliest stages. After treatment ends, some women report fearing that every ache and pain is an indication that the cancer has returned or spread [156]. This can be difficult for family and friends to understand. They expect the survivor to be relieved that the cancer treatments are completed and ready to move on with her life. For many survivors, however, the possibility of recurrence and further treatment is always in the back of their mind [157].

> "Every time my back aches or I have a headache, I think my cancer has spread in my body. I hate to go to the doctor because I just know that one of these days he will tell me that my cancer is back."

Survivors who receive a diagnosis of recurrence can experience a number of emotions upon hearing that their cancer has returned, including fear, anger, and guilt [157]. They may fear the unknown outcome of their newest diagnosis or be afraid that the cancer may have spread to other parts of the body. They may feel angry at God for forcing them to face cancer again, or angry at their own body for betraying them by getting sick again. Some survivors may even feel guilty that something they did, or did not do, during their first cancer experience caused the disease to return. In these ways, the news that cancer has returned can often be more emotionally devastating than the original diagnosis.

> "The first time I was diagnosed with cancer I was a poster-child for a positive attitude. I was sure I had beaten my cancer and survived! When the cancer returned several years later, I was devastated. I'm no longer positive and I have faced the fact that the cancer won and I'm going to die."

Survivors who learn that their cancer has metastasized from the original site face a unique set of challenges. The learning curve is shifted back for these survivors, as they must try to understand the vocabulary and nature of their new diagnosis. Cancer behaves differently in different parts of the body, so treatment options and survival rates will vary depending on the site and the stage of the metastasized cancer. It can be especially difficult for survivors who receive a second cancer diagnosis while they are still undergoing treatment for a primary cancer. They can feel that they have lost any sense of control of the outcome of their cancer or that the physical and financial costs of treatment have been futile.

Regardless of where survivors are in their cancer journey when they receive a diagnosis of recurrence, there are important things to keep in mind that may help them to remain optimistic. First and foremost, survivors should be reminded that their previous treatments failed them; they did not fail the treatment [157]. Survivors should be able to focus on moving forward with their current treatment, instead of needlessly blaming themselves for the outcome of past treatment efforts. Similarly, survivors should keep in mind that cancer treatments are continuously evolving, which means that less aggressive but equally effective treatment options might be available that did not exist the first time they faced a cancer diagnosis. The same is true for the management of side effects, which many cancer survivors say are worse than the treatment itself.

> "The treatments feel worse than death, but every treatment means more time with my kids and family. I will do anything for more time."

Survivors should also remember that they have developed coping mechanisms from their previous diagnosis and treatment. If they question their ability to cope with a recurrence, it may be helpful for them to reflect on the sources of strength they discovered after their first diagnosis. Reminding them that they are already survivors may help them rediscover and refine previous coping strategies to help them through the challenges of cancer recurrence [157].

The communication of distressing news is demanding for both the doctor and survivor [158,159]. Disclosure of a short life expectancy has been specifically identified by both clinicians and survivors as an important and contentious issue [160,161]. Previously, the debate about the issue was focused on whether or not to tell the patient the prognosis. However, in more recent times, researchers are concerned with what information to give and how to convey it [162].

"I was told on the phone that it was now in my spine and I knew I was going to die. My life was over."

Research demonstrates that a clear majority of cancer survivors in the Western world prefer detailed information about their disease and expected outcome, although information needs can vary across different phases of the illness [74,162-164]. Legal rulings have emphasized the responsibility of doctors to provide all necessary information in some jurisdictions. Nevertheless, survivors often misunderstand the status of their disease and the aim of treatment and commonly overestimate their life expectancy [162]. A clear understanding of their condition and treatment is particularly important for advanced cancer survivors because treatment may have side effects that significantly reduce quality of life [165].

Issues that concern clinicians about communicating life expectancy to patients include how much information to give, the difficulties with prognostication, and how to disclose prognostic uncertainty without increasing anxiety, reducing trust, and destroying hope [74,160,162,166,167]. Others believe that expressing this prognostic ambiguity carefully to patients is one means of engendering hope and that providing information decreases anxiety associated with ignorance and uncertainty [162,168]. However, doctors commonly find these interactions challenging. The best way of presenting prognostic information to optimize understanding, psychological adjustment, and decision-making is uncertain. To date, much of the communication literature has focused on how to break bad news, and there is little guidance available for clinicians in estimating or communicating prognosis, particularly in the context of newly diagnosed metastatic disease.

"My doctor wants me to call in hospice, but I'm not ready to give up yet. If I call in hospice, I will just die and I'm not ready to give up yet."

The literature suggests that cancer survivors frequently misunderstand much of what they are told, incorrectly state the extent of their disease and the goal of treatment, and overestimate their prognosis [160,162,163]. Such misunderstanding may lead survivors to make decisions contrary to their best interests, for example choosing futile life-extending therapy at the expense of quality of life. This misunderstanding commonly reported by cancer survivors may be attributed in part to poor communication by physicians. Although most doctors in the Western world now report their diagnosis to cancer patients, discussing a poor prognosis is often more difficult [162].

> "I am just holding out for the miracle cure. They could discover a cure for cancer in the next year, so I need to try every drug possible just to hold on until they might find a cure. I think the drugs are going to kill me before the cancer."

Doctors face particular difficulties when discussing life expectancy with patients with a "poor" prognosis. Such information raises immediate issues for the patient, and the information required includes much shorter time frames than the long range forecasting required in early stage disease. Considerable inaccuracy in doctors' predictions of the survival of individual patients with incurable disease has been documented [169]. In addition, physicians often have difficulties in providing hope and discussing prognosis with metastatic cancer patients. For example, Bradley and colleagues reviewed medical records of randomly selected terminally ill cancer patients from six treatment centers in the US in 2001 and found the discussions about prognosis were documented in only 38% of patient files [170].

> "My doctor told me to get my affairs in order, but when I asked what that means …. He just said it means get your affairs in order! I didn't know if he was telling me I was going to die in a week, month or years."

Discussing end-of-life is also difficult for survivors and their families because they fear it means "giving up", and that the medical team will stop trying to cure them. Oncology social workers are becoming increasingly important in supporting survivors, their families, and physicians in engaging in conversations about end-of-life plans. In a qualitative study, end-of-life oncology patients desired the opportunity to prepare themselves and their family for the end of life, to complete unfinished business, and to achieve a sense of peace before they died [171]. They also wanted health care team members with whom they could discuss goals of end of life and be instrumental to them in this process [171]. The medical team is often unprepared at how to address end-of-life goals and the importance of quality of life.

> "My doctor suggested that I contact hospice, but I didn't want to do that because it means that everyone is giving up hope on me. I still have hope!"

Training is needed in palliative care to address the psychosocial and spiritual needs of advanced survivors. One example of training provided to oncology social workers is the National Cancer Institute funded ACE Project (Advocating for Clinical Excellence: Transdisciplinary Palliative Care Education). The ACE Project was designed to offer enhanced leadership and advocacy education to selected psycho-oncology professionals [172]. Many social workers work in hospice settings providing end-of-life care to oncology patients. Despite efforts to increase understanding of the role of hospice, many survivors, especially minority and underserved survivors, underutilize these services. Oncology social workers are in a unique position to train other health care professionals on the needs of end-of-life patients and to educate about quality of life issues during this phase of care and make timely referrals to palliative and hospice care.

Chapter 5

HEALTH CARE IN THE UNITED STATES

"Society has left us no choice. Either you pay or you die, because without insurance the doctors are not going to see you."

Access to quality health care is an essential part of a woman's cancer experience and survival. Thus, it is important to understand the evolution of our health care system and how the current system impacts the lives of cancer survivors.

"A lot of doctors won't see you without insurance. The first question they ask is what kind of insurance do you have?"

DOMESTIC HEALTH CARE TO A HEALTH CARE INDUSTRY

Prior to the 18th century, health care in the United States was referred to as "domestic medicine" centering on family care. It was usually performed by women and utilized home remedies. By the end of the century, medical training became more standardized and physicians became more prevalent. By 1900, health care had transformed from a familial approach to an industrialized approach. The number of hospitals went from a couple of hundred to over 4,000, and health care now played a major factor in American economic culture. As the turn of the 19th century approached, our country moved from a largely rural agricultural nation to an urban mass-production environment, causing social inequities to emerge.

Between 1900 and 1915, over 15 million immigrants came to the United States. This time span is referred to as the Progressive Era, when many middle-class white Americans voiced concerns about the potential threats associated with fast paced industrialization and urbanization. Municipalities were ill equipped to provide the necessary infrastructure for their rapidly growing towns. Rural health facilities were least prepared and offered limited or inadequate medical care. Progressive reformers, both individually and collectively, began to look at social issues such as labor protection, health care services and access, urban living and environmental protections.

In 1901, the American Medical Association (AMA) began to gain strength as a powerful national force. The AMA grew from 8,000 physician members in 1900 to over 70,000 in 1910. This time is considered the beginning of "organized medicine", when physicians were no longer expected to provide free medical care at hospitals, and the first national conference was held on "social insurance." At the same time, social reformers argued for labor and health reforms. Reformers believed that social medicine would open access to medical care for all citizens, regardless of social class. This new order of social medicine was seen as a right of citizenship and was grounded in the premise that the health of a collective was a stake in the health status of each individual [173]. As expectations grew for a just and moral society, reformers fought for a balance between increased industry and working conditions, housing, education, and health care.

To address many of the social issues of the time, progressive reformers took decisive actions to protect the fast growing immigrant population that made up most of the urban poor. Most notably was the establishment of "social settlements" in urban tenement neighborhoods that provided greater access to health care, vocational training, and child care. Soon the social settlement movement could be seen throughout the nation's largest cities. Jane Addams was instrumental in moving social thought to the belief that it was the wealthy who had a moral obligation to improve society for those more vulnerable and less fortunate [174].

HEALTH CARE 1900 – 1950

In 1901, after President McKinley's assassination, Theodore Roosevelt became president and brought the Progressive agenda to the White House. Roosevelt proposed several pieces of legislation meant to protect the health and welfare of the people. With Roosevelt as president, the help of the Progressive movement, and the fast-paced advancement of technology, a shift occurred in the perception of government's responsibility to the well-being and safety of its people. Citizens looked to government and employers to provide safe work environments and health care regardless of social class. In 1911 the first workers compensation law was passed, protecting employees by regulating sticker oversight and maintenance of machinery, and forming a social welfare for employees injured or killed on the job. Throughout Roosevelt's tenure as president, legislation was passed and government regulations put in place to protect society against unscrupulous business practices and abusive employers. Nonetheless, little progress was made in improving health care access and quality to all the nation's citizens. This may have been due in large part to the United States' entry into the war in 1917.

Eventually, local physicians and large employers took on the role of addressing the many labor health care needs and problems associated with the rural and urban poor. In 1929, Dr. Michael Shadid started the first rural farmer's cooperative health plan in Elk City, Oklahoma, for approximately 6,000 people. Dr. Shadid sold shares at $50 to anyone in the county willing to invest in the first cooperatively owned and managed hospital in the nation. In return for their $50 investment, they received health care at a reduced rate. In the same year, Baylor University Hospital in Dallas, Texas teamed up with the Dallas school district to organize what is considered to be the first real group insurance plan. Over 1,500 teachers were given access to 21 days of hospital care per year in exchange for an annual payment of $6. This plan eventually evolved into the company known as Blue Cross. With the success of this insurance arrangement, similar prepaid arrangements soon were being negotiated with physicians, creating Blue Shield. It was in these early days of prepaid medical services that Health Maintenance Organizations (HMOs) emerged.

During World War II, Henry Kaiser funded the first workers compensation, clinic-based system. In 1937, he provided comprehensive health care services to his workers and their families who were building an aqueduct in southern California to transport water from the Colorado River to Los Angles. A similar program was started in 1942 at Kaiser's shipyards and steel mills. Kaiser worked with Dr. Sidney Garfield to build an infrastructure that focused on prevention as well as injury and illness [175]. For five cents a day, workers had access to health coverage and for an additional five cents workers could receive health coverage for non-work related injuries. After WWII, Kaiser offered a similar prepaid health coverage plan to the public. The AMA worked fiercely to erode support for the up-and-coming prepaid plans and cooperatives by ostracizing participating physicians from referrals, consultations, and admitting privileges to hospitals. Eventually the AMA was found guilty of violating the Sherman Antitrust Act. Despite AMA's attempt, the Kaiser Permanente was founded and now provides health care to over 8 million members. Kaiser Permanente is considered the first true Health Management Organization (HMO) [176].

It was not until Franklin D. Roosevelt, the fifth cousin of Theodore Roosevelt, was elected president that government re-engaged in a national debate on employment-based health care. During WWII, the federal government, under FDR, supported the idea of employment based health insurance by allowing employers (not employees) to deduct the cost of health care as an operating expense and by exempting employer health insurance from taxes, thereby connecting health insurance with employment. As the nation faced the longest economic collapse in modern history during the Great Depression, more than 15 million Americans (one-fourth) lost their jobs. It was a time of social and economic uncertainty that threatened the health of the nation.

In 1934, President Roosevelt created the President's Committee on Economic Security (CES) to make recommendations on a national program that would protect its citizens against disease, promote access and quality of medical care, and protect against economic insecurity caused by an illness or disability. The committee reviewed issues concerning social welfare, unemployment, child health care and poverty among the elderly; however, this committee omitted studying a social insurance plan for fear that the AMA would oppose all social services in a protest against a public health care plan. President Roosevelt continued to hold and speak out on the ideology that government must safeguard democracy and political stability by promoting social justice and equality, an ideological framework he outlined in "The Economic Bill of Rights."

The national debate around the topic of a comprehensive health care plan continued in 1945 with President Truman. He gave a speech proposing that the federal government should play a key role in the health care of the nation and introduced the first single- payer system design that would include all Americans. Truman's proposal was similar to FDR's, but emphasized the expansion of public health services and medical research. Key health care design elements of his "Fair Deal" included reducing financial barriers, improving access, expanding disability compensation and a nation-wide system of health insurance.

President Truman's quest for universal health care was largely defeated by critics linking his ideas to a socialist and communist government. Opposition, once again, from the APA framed the reform debate as an increase in big government lowered competition, increased medical fees, inefficiency and a decrease in quality. Despite the fear of the spread of communism during the early days of the Cold War, and the AMA's $5 million plan to denounce Truman's plan, there was a populous agreement on a health care system funded and controlled by the federal government. An important fact to keep in mind was the health of the nation's economy. It was a time of prosperity, unlike the hard times under FDR, and the need for health care reform seemed less urgent.

BIRTH OF MANAGED CARE 1960 – 2000

For the next twenty years, prepaid health care plans grew slowly and the employee-based model proved to be risky. In the 1950s over half of the population, mainly from the middle class, had some type of health care insurance. The other half without any form of health insurance was largely made up of the poor and elderly. Not much happened in terms of national health insurance initiatives in the 1950s under President Eisenhower. The nation focused more on unions as a vehicle for health insurance. In the early prepaid models of HMOs, physicians were treated and paid as hospital staff models. In the mid-1960s, however, Independent Physician Associations (IPAs) were developed, creating a new health care market. IPAs are made up of individuals or groups of physicians who directly contract with hospitals on a fee-for-service reimbursement structure. The inherent problem with fee-for-service arrangements is the potential for over utilization of medical services.

The term "HMO" was officially coined in the early 1970s during the Nixon administration to encompass an organized health care system that is responsible for the financing and delivery of medical services [176]. In most situations, an HMO is a combination of a health insurer and a health care delivery system. With broad support for the concept of HMOs, there came less political discussions on socializing medicine and a universal health plan. President Nixon, along with strong support from Congress, passed the HMO Act of 1973, which required employers with over 25 employees to offer at least one HMO to all employees. The Act set federal standards for HMOs and then provided low cost growth and development loans. In addition, the HMO Act brought accountability and health promotion strategies where they were needed the most, in rural America. The development and passage of the HMO Act was in response to a perceived national health care crisis originating in the late 1960s and early 1970s. Health care costs rose sharply over this period, leading many in the industry to believe the way to manage "out-of-control" spending was to coordinate care through a delivery system focused on preventive care, increased access to quality care, managed utilization, shared risk among stakeholders and outcome based research.

This new health care delivery system brought a sense of shared responsibility between the stakeholders. Physicians and hospitals that had been reimbursed under a fee-for-service arrangement with little or no cost or utilization controls were now held financially responsible for the services they rendered when they contracted with HMOs. Despite, the "pushback" from many group practices, several successful HMOs legitimized the movement with strong member enrollment. HMOs were originally designed as non-profit entities, but in the early 1980s for-profit HMOs began to proliferate along with other managed health care strategies. In 1981, only 12% of the market was served by for-profit HMOs compared to approximately 65% in 1997 [177].

The new for-profit HMOs drastically changed the way health care was administered in America. The stakeholders of the once non-for-profit health care industry found themselves under regulatory and competitive pressures. During this time, physicians lost their autonomy, HMO enrollment grew as the federal government moved Medicare and Medicaid members into HMOs, large employers switched their premium based health benefits into HMOs, and consumers began to complain about limited access to their preferred choice of physicians. It was at this time that several new strategies emerged to meet varying degrees of the public need and expectations.

The first of the new strategies were preferred provider networks (PPOs). PPOs are different than HMOs in two respects. First, PPOs allow enrollees to choose providers of care outside contracted networks, but with higher out of pocket expenses, such as deductibles. Secondly, PPOs do not accept any financial risk; rather, risks remain with employers and insurance companies (payers). In response to the flexible PPOs, points of service organizations (PSOs) were established to manage utilization. The PSOs acted as an intermediate between HMOs and PPOs by placing a gatekeeper, such as a primary care physician, to manage utilization of services through a referral process. Eventually, HMOs integrated with hospitals and physician groups to form physician-hospital organizations (PHOs) [178].

As an outgrowth of these new strategies, "utilization review" emerged as the new buzz word. This goal of this review process was to coordinate care for the purposes of improving continuity and quality of care and to lower costs. Utilization review is often times referred to as case management and is considered the bedrock of managed care. Managed care is a nebulous concept that combines methods of organizing health care service delivery and reimbursement.

THE UPS AND DOWNS OF MANAGED CARE

Enrollment into HMOs grew from 30 million in 1989 to 56 million people by 1995 and over 80 million in 1999. The growth of HMOs was due to private employers contracting with managed care companies to help control their growing health care expenses. By promising to hold down cost while providing quality care, managed care organizations were somewhat successful in their promise. Managed care strategies helped reduce double digit health care premium increases of the 1980s to a 2% increase in the mid 1990s. By 1995, over 70% of the nations HMOs were for-profit, and over half of all individuals who had job-related health care insurance were enrolled in some type of a managed care plan.

"In the beginning, I was a strong advocate of the managed care philosophy of promoting preventative medicine and improving access to quality care while being fiscal responsible. My healthcare career began with a start-up for-profit managed care company. I remember working long hours and weekends to ensure the company offered quality service plans that were comprehensive and integrated. As the company service lines grew, so did the company's profit and officer's compensation. I watched for years how our once well intended services became more restrictive as the company's focus moved away from preventative medicine and access to quality care and more towards a profit driven philosophy. At first hand I witnessed collaborative relationships between hospitals, physicians and payers disintegrate due to never ending conflicts of interest and a growing public concern with managed care organization's true intent. I remember negotiating aggressively low reimbursement rates with small providers of care (i.e., Home Health), which supported the company's focus on cost containment, only to have them file for bankruptcy in 2 years. Finally, I want to say that I think the philosophy behind the managed care design is the right one, I just think it was poorly executed".

James Robinson, in *The End of Managed Care,* frames the downfall of managed care as an "economic success but a political failure" [179]. This process was frustrating and disappointing to all those involved in the process. According to Robinson, the dichotomous relationship between consumerism and corporate dominance became a strategy of giving with one hand and taking away with the other [179]. On one hand, managed care promised comprehensive benefits; yet, on the other hand, it restricted many of those benefits through utilization reviews. In response to the dissatisfaction of employees because of limited choices in providers, hospitals, and services, employers moved from tightly managed HMOs to less restrictive plans, such as PPOs and PSOs [179]. Moving from a market-driven system into a consumer-driven system, which offered more choice and more personal control, came with a high price tag to the consumer. In both scenarios, low income consumers suffer the greatest loss. Under tightly controlled HMOs, low income consumers faced systemic barriers to care, whereas, under the current consumer-driven system they are unable to afford the out-of-pocket expenses associated with choice.

CURRENT HEALTH CARE TRENDS

Health care costs remain the fastest growing employer expense in the United States. To shoulder the rising cost, employers are forced to off-set the expense by passing much of the increase to their employees through higher premiums and co-payments. In 2007, the 9.3 million individuals participating in an employer health insurance plan saw their premiums increased by at least 6.1%, two times the rate of inflation [180]. Employees utilizing their employer health insurance plans, on a whole, are paying $1,400 more in premiums annually for family coverage than they did in 2000 [181]. According to the Kaiser Family Foundation, premiums for employer-related health insurance have risen four times faster than the average employee salary since 2000. The 1.3 million people having non-group coverage are three times more likely to incur higher financial burdens than any other group. Others at risk of incurring higher than average financial burdens are minorities, the poor, low-income, non-elderly individuals with disabilities, people suffering from a chronic illness, or those living in rural environments [182].

Economists with the Office of Management and Budget (OMB) have found that rising health care costs directly impact an employer's ability to offer affordable health insurance coverage to their employees. Consequently, employers reduce or are forced to eliminate health benefits. As a result, public programs such as Medicare and Medicaid continue to grow at a faster rate than private pay insurance programs.

An estimated 50 million people under the age of 65 and living in families spend, on an average, more than ten percent of their household income on health care. Families spending ten percent or more of their household income are considered to be underinsured [183]. In 2003, an estimated 17.1 million people under the age of 65 were underinsured, including 9.3 million people receiving employment-related coverage, 1.3 million having private non-group coverage, and 6.6 million people enrolled in some type of public health care plan [182].

Historically, the health care debate in this nation has been more about access and insurance than on the actual practice of medicine. The federal government's involvement in health care will only increase over the next decade as the nation's population ages and becomes more diverse, and costs soar. The notion of universal health care coverage seems to be gaining support among policy makers. With the shift towards universal healthcare, the current acute care model would move more towards preventative medicine, whereby containing the high costs associated with chronic illnesses. Despite the current vigor around a single payer system, history has proven that this national debate is far from being over. Meanwhile, states like California and Massachusetts have passed laws that require all residents to have a minimum level of coverage and provide subsidies for low-income families. Roadblocks to health coverage based on pre-existing conditions, genetics, and ability to pay for services must be eliminated from our health care system.

> "Once you've had cancer – breast cancer, or whatever type cancer it is – if you trying to get into another insurance. Forget that."

As the federal and state governments move slowly towards universal care, employers remain the backbone of our health insurance system. The future role of employer based insurance is unclear. One thing is certain, the current health care system falls short in providing access to quality care for all women diagnosed with cancer. The health care system is difficult to understand and sometimes impossible to negotiate. Minority and underserved cancer survivors need social workers to help them navigate through the health care system.

> "From January to May I was without insurance – a private paying patient. Every doctor I saw – radiation – had to be paid for in cash, because I didn't have insurance. I don't have any money left. I don't know what to do."

Oncology social workers should provide survivors with resources to help them negotiate with their insurance companies, such as *What Cancer Survivors Need to Know about Health Insurance* by Calder and Pollitz (available in English and Spanish). The U.S. has the ability to provide the highest quality treatment in the world, but unfortunately, many women never get access to the quality of care they deserve. Oncology social workers have the skills and expertise to advocate for women and their families as they struggle to get access to quality care.

> "I felt lost and overwhelmed with all the different doctors and all the insurance stuff. It was worse than the cancer. I didn't know where to turn for help. I owe so much money that I just cry all the time. My kids have nothing now."

At the state and national level, social workers need to lobby for a health care system that provides treatment based on a patient's diagnosis, not financial constraints.

Chapter 6

FINANCIAL BURDEN OF CANCER

"This disease isn't supposed to make you homeless ….. but I'm going to be on the street with my kids in the next few months. It's just not right!"

In 2007, the National Center for Health Statistics reported health care costs in the U.S. exceeded the nation's expenditures on national defense by 4.3%, representing 2.3 trillion dollars and are projected to reach 4.2 trillion by 2016. Although the U.S. spends more on health care than other industrialized countries, the same report suggested that over 47 million people are currently uninsured. When compared to other industrialized countries in 2005, the U.S. spent 16% of its gross domestic product (GDP) on health care, while health care costs in Switzerland accounted for 10.9% of their GDP, in Germany 10.7%, in Canada 9.7% and in France 9.5%. Each of these countries, with the exception of the U.S., provides health insurance to all their citizens. According to the Agency for Health Care Research and Quality [182], health care costs accounted for 7% of GDP for the U.S. in the 1960s, but expenditures had increased to 9.1% in 1980 and 13.6% by 1997. Health care costs have grown at a faster rate than the U.S. economy for many years.

According to the American Cancer Society [40], cancer is the most costly illness in the U.S., exceeding $219 billion in 2007, including $89 billion in direct medical costs and $18.2 billion in lost productivity. In addition to the physical suffering experienced by individuals diagnosed with cancer, there are considerable financial hardships and access barriers to quality health care. Cancer patients with health coverage often find their premiums and out-of-pocket expenses continuing to rise after a cancer diagnosis. One study found that over 28% of individuals diagnosed with cancer have a total burden exceeding 10% of their family income, and 11.4% of families spend in excess of 20% [184]. In the same study, one-third of families dealing with a cancer diagnosis lost most or all of their savings, while one-fifth of the families had a member quit work to care for the cancer survivor. On an average, individuals with health care coverage through a federally-funded program or a private plan saw an increase in out-of-pocket expenses, rising 56% from 1996 ($464) to 2003 ($834).

The ACS has shown that individuals with inadequate or no health insurance coverage are less likely to receive recommended cancer screening, more likely to be diagnosed at a later stage, and have lower survival rates. As a result, this population requires more service utilization for longer periods of time. Uninsured patients are 1.6 times more likely to die in five years from a cancer diagnosis than those with private insurance. Individuals with private health insurance are twice as likely to have had mammography or colorectal cancer screening.

Private or employer-related health insurance does not always transcend socio-demographic factors such as race, ethnicity, education, income or economic status. The literature suggests that low income, ethnic minorities are less likely to receive quality care, even after controlling for socioeconomic status [185,186].

HEALTH CARE AND ECONOMIC DISPARITIES

In 2003, the National Center for Health Statistics estimated 33% of the U.S. populations belonged to a racial or ethnic minority group, and that number is projected to exceed 50% by 2050. Underserved population groups are 10 times less likely to receive timely medical care than their counterparts. In 2007, the National Health Care Disparities Report investigated the quality and utilization of health care in America among different racial, ethnic, and socioeconomic subgroups and found three key themes [187]:

1. Overall, disparities in health care quality and access are not getting smaller.
2. Progress is being made, but many of the biggest gaps in quality and access have not been reduced.
3. The persistent problem of no insurance is a major barrier to reducing disparities.

A large household survey between 1996 and 2003 that targeted adults younger than 65 living in a family (two or more), identified several national trends between a family's insurance status, their total health care costs, and financial burden [184]. Underinsured has been defined as a family spending 10% or more of their household income on health care [183]. Based on this definition, the analysis found three subgroups consistently at risk: families having employment-related coverage but considered underinsured, families insured by a public program, and the uninsured. In 2003, 5.5% of the 9.3 million individuals considered underinsured spent in excess of 10% of their family income on health care, while 2.1 % spent over 20% of their income. Furthermore, 19.4% of individuals covered by a public program faced financial burdens exceeding 10% of their family income and 10.7% of individuals faced more than a 20% burden. Findings from this analysis provide evidence that financial burdens related to health care rose across the study population as a whole and that the poor and the uninsured faced the largest burdens [184].

> "I have insurance, but I still don't have money for the co-pay. I don't have a job or money to buy food."

Women who have public insurance through a federally-funded program spent more in out-of-pocket expenses ($4,678) than women with private health coverage ($2,460) and not surprisingly, women with no insurance ($1,512) spent the least [188]. Among the poor and the uninsured, a simple $15 copayment may be a deterrent for many seeking health care services and an even greater deterrent for those seeking preventative health services such as cancer screenings. For some, this financial burden may require choosing between health care and other necessities of life. For all choosing to address the necessities of life, they inadvertently create additional barriers to the prevention, early detection, and treatment needed to reduce cancer disparities.

"They're saying, "You've got to pay something on them....Or we won't treat you anymore...'$10.... $10.' They say, 'You can pay $10.' They going to call you every day...Every day until you send that $10 – until they receive it...But they don't understand, with no income...With no income – how you going to get $10?...They expect you to borrow the money from somebody, so if you borrow the money, how you going to pay them back?"

UNEQUAL ACCESS AND CARE

Literature provides evidence that women with private insurance have significantly better rates of survival than women with other insurance statuses. For example, minority women insured by Medicaid are more likely to be undertreated for breast cancer once they are diagnosed [97,189]. The medically underserved, regardless of insurance status, experience difficulties in accessing medical care throughout the continuum of cancer care. It has been reported that women enrolled in a Medicaid program and those having no insurance were at a higher risk of not receiving post breast-conserving surgery (BCS) radiation therapy and/or systematic chemotherapy. Findings also suggest uninsured women were less likely to receive radiation therapy after BCS, and women insured by Medicaid were less likely to receive chemotherapy when compared to women with private insurance [61].

"I didn't have any insurance. And I didn't know who to turn to. I have 4th stage breast cancer. Before I found out, I kept asking my doctor for a mammogram for like 3 or 4 years and they wouldn't give me one because they said I was too young. When they finally did something about the lumps, it was too late because it had already spread all over my body."

On one hand, studies have also found that women with no history of previous cancer and private insurance are more likely to undergo aggressive evaluations than minority women with public or no insurance coverage [53,54]. In contrast, others have found that low-income women covered under a federally-funded screening program receive similar standards of care to that of all women studied [190,191]. Most studies agree, however, that low income women with early stage breast cancer are less likely to receive radiation therapy and have a longer time interval to treatment when compared to other women.

"I'm on Medicare and asked for a second opinion. My doctor asked, "Why are you going after a second opinion? I already told you everything."...the type of insurance you have seems to dictate the type of treatment you get..."

Coburn and colleagues used a cohort of 6,876 invasive breast cancer cases from Rhode Island's Cancer Registry (RICR) to investigate if there was a correlation between treatment and insurance status. The study supports earlier findings that insurance status is significantly associated with treatment. Furthermore, women with Medicaid, Medicare and no insurance are more likely to present to treatment with larger tumors and are less likely to receive reconstructive surgery when compared to women with private health insurance [192].

When considering age and gender, older individuals (55 to 64 years) are more likely to incur a financial burden, and women across all ages are more likely to incur higher financial health burdens than men the same age. Regardless of insurance status, age, and gender, the burden of illness has increasingly caused financial difficulty as evidenced in bankruptcy studies [193]. Bankruptcy studies indicate that medical expenses and loss of job related to a medical illness or disability are often cited in the top three reasons for filing bankruptcy.

THE COST OF CANCER

Empirical evidence shows that the absence of health insurance causes financial instability and in some cases, for low income families, impoverishment.

> "My biggest concern was the money that I would pay for my treatment, not the disease itself."

In a review of health insurance policies and costs, Arozullah and colleagues found significant gaps in covered medical services for breast cancer patients. For those individuals with health care coverage with a federally funded program or a private plan and having a breast cancer diagnosis, out-of-pocket expenses and lost income averaged $1,455 per month. Over 40% reported spending more than $500 a month on out-of-pocket expenses, and a third reported spending between $1,000 and $5,000 a month [194].

> "I'm about to get put out. Probably the end of the month… because I had to pay my light bill… and you got to feed the kids…you have to stay at the shelter before you get Section 8 housing."

Current research provides information on cost and expenditures associated with direct and indirect medical and non-medical expenditures for cancer patients. Little is known about the cost associated with care giving in terms of out-of-pocket expenses and lost wages experienced by the caregiver. Less is known about long-term social and health care costs associated with minority women diagnosed with cancer. Most noteworthy are the varying degrees in which researchers define and measure such costs. Therefore, estimates regarding the different types of costs associated with cancer should be interpreted with caution. Regardless of insurance status, the financial burden of all types of cancer is disproportionately greatest among women living in the lowest levels of household income.

> "It makes you homeless. You work for years, years, and years and just because you get sick you lose everything. It just isn't fair!"

In a self-reported assessment on the financial burden of cancer for 156 women diagnosed with breast cancer who had insurance, researchers found that out-of-pocket expenses accounted for 41% of their total burden accounting for a monthly mean of $597 [194]. The most commonly reported out-of-pocket or direct medical expenses were medications (80%), physician visits (66%), alternative or complimentary health aides (48%), and hospital bills (45%). Even a small co-pay may result in missed or delayed treatment for some women.

> "And if you don't have your co-pay, a lot of times they say, "Well, we can reschedule. When is best for you?" meaning 'when you have the money you can come back'."

The financial burden of cancer is often overwhelming, especially for those who are uninsured or underinsured. This financial burden is often the most overwhelming aspect of the cancer experience.

"I have cancer, I am homeless. That's not fair. That's just not right."

Women and their families are faced with medical bills and other expenses. Indirect costs associated with an illness or disease are defined in terms of lost time from work, cost associated with caregivers, disability, and premature retirement or death. Such costs should include all expenditures experienced by the patient, family members and anyone caring for the patient. Most cost analyses only calculate expenditures experienced by the patient. However, Arozullah and colleagues found that indirect costs accounted for half of the patient's monthly financial burden, with an average cost of $727.

"I owe over $1,000. They call everyday and say "You've got to pay something, or we won't treat you anymore."

Additionally, these women missed an average of seven hours per week at work, and 62% reduced their hours of work after their cancer diagnosis. For low-income, head of household women this loss can interfere with their ability to pay for childcare, co-payments or transportation [194].

"I wiped out my savings taking care of me. My son paid when I no longer had a savings. I thought I was saving to retire early, but I didn't realize that it was going to be paid to save my life. This is sad, but society has left us with no choice .... Either you pay or you die! Now my son and I are both without any savings!"

Even among people with health care insurance, many are inadequately covered for a cancer diagnosis and are at risk of a health-related financial burden. For those individuals without any insurance or who belong to a minority group, the risk is exponentially greater. The impact of health insurance status on the access and quality of care someone receives and the disproportionate out-of-pocket expenses low-income families bear has been *business as usual* for much too long. For low-income women, their lack of insurance or being underinsured may mean missed, delayed, or fewer treatment opportunities. Literature and research have clearly provided the consequential effects of such actions in the mortality rate for these women.

Chapter 7

PRACTICAL CONCERNS

"The social worker approached me and asked "Anything you want me to do for you?" Yes ... pay bills, help me talk to the doctor, fix my insurance problems, rent? Well, she just wanted to talk about my problems NOT solve them, so I didn't call her anymore."

Direct, nonmedical expenses include such items as childcare, housekeeping, home care, wigs, prostheses, over-the-counter medications and expenses associated with travel. For those individuals who have health insurance, non-medical items are rarely covered. Cancer insurance and long-term insurance policies are available and help reduce the unforeseen out-of-pocket expenses that create financial burdens for many families who have health insurance. However, health insurance supplements are only beneficial to the population that can afford to pay the additional premiums.

"I had insurance, but not enough."

CHILDCARE

Whether the woman works outside the home in addition to raising her children, or she looks after her children full time, cancer will most likely affect her and her family's normal routines. Cancer treatments such as surgery and chemotherapy often bring with them exhaustion, and a woman who, pre-illness, found the duties of caring for her children manageable might now be in a position where she is simply too fatigued to look after her children. Feelings of guilt and inadequacy about her perceived change in ability can be overwhelming, but it is important for mothers with cancer to know that they can ask for help with their children.

A break from childcare responsibilities is welcome and needed for any mother, and mothers with cancer may especially benefit from the chance to rest. Some mothers reported that their spouses and partners were helpful when it came to assisting with the childcare duties; however, others were left to fulfill the childcare responsibilities on their own.

"My husband didn't understand why I couldn't get things done at home. I didn't have much support at home."

Other sources of childcare can come in the form of friends and other family members. Often these people want to help the woman who has been diagnosed, and providing childcare is a tangible way in which they can do so. Hiring a nanny, bringing in the occasional babysitter, and enrolling children in daycare are more formal childcare options that are available.

It is important for the oncology social worker to discuss the difficulties of childrearing responsibilities and assist the survivor and her family in coming up with strategies to deal with the demands of children. Women often want to protect their children and keep their routine as "normal" as possible; however, this is often emotionally and physically draining for the survivor.

> "All I want to do is spend time with my kids and play like we used to, but the good days go by so quickly. Most days I feel too sick to play with my kids. I feel like I'm missing out on so much that they are doing."

It is necessary to develop a realistic plan with mothers to meet both the needs of their children as well as their need to take care of themselves.

TRANSPORTATION

Transportation to and from treatment centers and doctor's appointments is often a major concern for cancer survivors. They are frequently too sick to drive themselves or may not have their own transportation. Waiting on public transportation can be very uncomfortable and emotionally stressful.

> "Nothing is better than having someone you know take you to treatment instead of being in van with a bunch of strangers. You might get off that machine at 3:00, but the van doesn't get there until 4:00. Then you have to ride all around and take everybody else home before you finally get home."

A lack of transportation can also result in missed treatments and missed appointments. Women sometimes feel uncomfortable to have to rely on family or friends to drive them to and from appointments.

> "When I was taking treatment my car broke down. I didn't have any way to get to the center. My aunt finally called the ACS, and they gave me a bus card. I was very thankful because I didn't know what to do."

It is important to assess women's practical support for things like driving to and from treatment visits. This practical support is very different than having someone to talk to about their feelings or concerns.

> "My family and friends offer to drive me to the treatment center and wait for me to finish my treatment, but I just hate to ask them to do that. It can sometimes be all day and people get tired of helping out for such a long period of time. Sometimes I feel so sick that I can barely make it home."

Often a woman's support system will be working during the day and not be able to assist with this type of help. Furthermore, public transportation is often unreliable or not available to women outside of urban areas. Transportation issues may be especially difficult for rural women traveling long distances for doctors' appointments and treatments. Oncology social workers need to continually assess the practical needs throughout the treatment phases because a woman's support system may change over time. In the beginning, women often have friends and family who volunteer to help with transportation, but as treatment continues for months and sometimes years, this support can become very limited or completely unavailable.

> "When I was first diagnosed, I had lots of people from church and my neighborhood offering to help, but after a year of treatment, most people just stop calling. My cancer is old news by now. I need more help now, but my support system has just about dried up. Thank goodness for my mom, but she is old and has a hard time driving. I'll probably die of a car wreck on the way to get treatment before the cancer kills me."

EMPLOYMENT

Cancer affects not only the survivor's ability to work during the treatment phase, but additionally survivors often face work limitations for years post-diagnosis.

> "I am trying to get disability. I can't work right now. Doctor's orders. I want to work. I have worked all my life."

Although various state and federal laws were enacted in the 1990s to provide some level of protection to cancer patients, these laws are not comprehensive and are subject to interpretation by the legal system [3]. Those women who depend on their jobs for survival are often those most likely to lose their jobs as a result of their cancer experience. These same women with lower paying jobs often do not have the resources to pursue their employment rights through the legal system.

> "I was still an employee, and when the doctor turned me loose to go back to work, that's when they wouldn't let me come back. I worked for 17 years... worked hard; worked smarter... they wouldn't let me come back."

Oncology social workers have a key role to play in educating women and their families about their rights as cancer survivors. Advocacy skills (as discussed later in this book) are key to empowering women to stand up for their rights within their work setting. It is also essential to provide resources on this topic, such as, *Working It Out: Your Employment Rights as a Cancer Survivor* by Barbara Hoffman (available in English and Spanish).

> "It is unfair to work on a job and then after you lose that job because you are sick you no longer have insurance. The job is gone and they take your insurance after all those years."

BODY IMAGE CONCERNS

Cancer treatment often brings with it loss of sense of femininity, loss of hair, and weight gain. These are changes that many women find difficult to face. Social norms that emphasize youth and beauty can make a woman especially sensitive to such changes in her appearance.

> 'The doctor walked in and said 'It's cancer' and then walked out. I had to wait from 11 to 3:30 until I could see the doctor. He said you have Stage 3 breast cancer. I asked if I would lose my hair and he said, 'What do you want your hair or your life'. I thought, 'I don't want that doctor' and I changed doctors.

Women have different views on other aspects of their bodies, such as breast conserving therapy or breast reconstruction. For some, this is an important part of recovery, but for others, it is more important to feel like they have "gotten all the cancer".

> "One of my main concerns was about my breasts being so big, I was going, "Am I going to have to walk around with one breast and look a certain way?" My appearance played a big deal in my battle."

It is important to talk to the women about the reasons motivating their treatment decisions. Body image is very personal and often not something that women are comfortable discussing with their treatment team, family, or friends.

Oncology social workers can play an important role in opening up the discussion about body image and how this is impacting treatment decisions and emotional adjustment.

> "At my age, I decided to have a double mastectomy to make sure I got it all, but if I had been younger I would have probably made a different choice."

PAIN AND FATIGUE

During and after treatment, many women suffer from pain and fatigue, which interferes with their ability to do even the most routine things. Pain is often a side effect of the cancer treatments, and approximately 70% of people with advanced cancer experience pain [195]. Although most pain can be managed or greatly eased with proper treatment, many women are not provided with adequate pain medication. African-Americans and Hispanics are less likely to receive the World Health Organization's recommended analgesics for pain compared to Caucasian patients [195]. Inadequate treatment of pain is more likely to occur in community oncology clinics that serve minority and low-income women. Studies have found that minority and underserved cancer patients do not call their health care provider about pain until it reaches a severe level, and that these patients are often not warned about the potential side effects of pain or how to manage their pain [195].

Fatigue is often more debilitating for women than the pain, and it is one of the most overlooked and undertreated side effects of cancer [196]. For some, the fatigue is mild and temporary during the treatment phase. For others, however, the fatigue is more severe and longer in duration – sometimes lasting months or years. Cancer-related fatigue (CRF) is defined as a persistent, subjective sense of tiredness related to cancer or cancer treatment that interferes with normal functioning [196]. CRF is not alleviated by rest and often interferes with a woman's ability to function in her daily life.

> "I get up in the morning long enough to feed my kids a bowl of cereal before school. I go back to bed and feel terrible all day. I try to get dressed at the end of the day right before they get off the bus. I feel terrible, but I try to put on a good face. I put them to bed at 7:00pm because I can't fake feeling good for more than a few hours. It takes all my energy just to get through those few hours with my kids. I don't want my kids to really know how bad I feel."

The exact causes of CRF are unknown. For some women, it may be the cancer itself, but for others, it may be more related to the cancer treatments. Women often describe a roller coaster cycle of fatigue with symptoms being worse at the beginning of the treatment cycle. CFR often results in decreased quality of life and increased levels of depression and emotional distress. CFR is also associated with loss of employment [196].

> "My treatment is finished and my family wants me to get back to normal. But, I feel tired and depressed all the time. I don't have any energy to do the things I used to love. I can hardly get through the day."

Pain and fatigue are not easily or routinely assessed in women with cancer. The diagnosis and treatment of pain and fatigue require open communication between the survivor and her treatment team. Both of these conditions rely on the patient to present her symptoms. However, women, especially minority and underserved women, often are reluctant to discuss these issues with their treatment team [196]. They think that the pain and fatigue are a normal part of the cancer experience. Oncology social workers need to work as part of the treatment team to ensure that women are discussing their pain and fatigue with their treatment team. It is important that oncology social workers assess women's level of fatigue and how this is interfering with their daily routine. This type of assessment should continue throughout the continuum of care because fatigue will often last for years after the treatment has ended.

OTHER CONCERNS

Cancer survivors are faced with numerous other issues and decisions that they are often unprepared to handle. Prior to a cancer diagnosis, many survivors were fulfilling numerous roles (e.g., mother, spouse, house manager, sole provider, employee, and caregiver of parents). A cancer diagnosis brings challenges to all of these roles and makes them difficult to manage.

> "My major concerns were my parents. I'm an only child and both my parents, at the time, were living and they were in their late 80s and 90s. I kept thinking what is going to happen to them if something happens to me? Who is going to care for them?"

Cancer survivors are also faced with difficult decisions to make about living wills, durable power of attorney for health care, wills, and trusts. These decisions are often overlooked by the health care treatment team, who is generally focused on disease management and symptom control.

> "My friend and I had many talks about where she wanted her ashes spread and what she wanted to happen when she was gone, but she never put those things in writing. She had no control over the progression of her cancer and no control over what happened to her body or her things when she died. I just wish she had put things into writing. She would be so disappointed to see what happened when she was gone. It was not her plan or wishes."

These issues are crucial for oncology social workers to address. One of the problems is when and who should discuss these with the survivor. Lack of a designated person to discuss these issues frequently results in them being overlooked or ignored by the health care team. The lack of clear direction on when these issues should be discussed often results in these issues not getting addressed until late stage, end-of-life, or not getting addressed at all. These issues should be discussed with cancer survivors early on in their diagnosis in order to give them time to prepare for their decisions. People often respond by saying "I don't need to do these things because I'm not going to die from cancer" or "I have several years before I need to think about those issues." It is important that the oncology social worker presents these issues to the survivor as vital steps to complete regardless of her cancer diagnosis. The oncology social worker may want to present these topics in the following ways:

> "I am glad that you are responding to your treatment in such a positive way and that you are doing much better. Before you complete your treatment, I would like to discuss a few important issues that all women should consider regardless of whether they have cancer or not. We just tend to not think about these issues until we're faced with something like a cancer diagnosis."

> "We are trying to get all women to do some long-term planning for themselves in the event of a health crisis or other emergency. We often don't think about issues such as wills and powers of attorney, until we are sick or something tragic happens. However, the best time to plan for these things is long before we actually need them. Have you ever talked or prepared an advanced directive or will, just in case something happens to you?

Chapter 8

DISTRESS IN CANCER PATIENTS

"You can't do anything but try to grasp whether the floor came out from under you or the sky fell down on top of you."

A review of the literature suggests that a diagnosis of cancer has the potential to result in significant emotional, physical and financial distress [3,197-204]. It is estimated that one-third of breast cancer patients experience significant distress and/or impairment of functioning in their lives [200,205,206]. In addition, this distress has been found to persist into long-term survivorship [207,208]. Despite the physical impact of cancer on an individual's health status, unmet psychosocial needs tend to compound the negative effects of the cancer survivors' experience.

"I think when you are diagnosed a lot of things go through your mind. It's just not one particular thing. It is your appearance, finances, am I going to live or die, and a lot of other things."

Women diagnosed with cancer report a significant increase in distress which may cause the development or progression of maladaptive coping skills early in their diagnosis and treatment [209]. Many studies have reported that distress is related to a woman's physical and psychological adjustment to cancer, which can be detrimental to decision making, treatment compliance and outcomes [80,197,210-218].

"A lot of people come up to me and say "You know, you've got a positive attitude. You're fighting this thing. I would've been bitter." I cry and I get this little sadness. But I think I've decided mine is more about – I'm experiencing the grief, the loss of my children. I'm losing them."

There is evidence to suggest that survivors experiencing isolation early in their diagnosis are at higher risk of developing and maintaining poor coping skills throughout their cancer experience [219,220].

"I never will forget – one of the patients – she was just having such a hard time, and she said, 'I can't look at myself in the mirror'. And I said, 'I look at myself in the mirror. I'm not a different person, and I have to keep telling myself I am the same person I was before this. You're going to have to do the same thing."

Distress can be present from the day of diagnosis into long-term survivorship. From the day of diagnosis, cancer survivors face life-altering decisions. The first few weeks after a diagnosis, vital treatment decisions are made and usually made with little knowledge and background. The concern in this primary phase is "information overload" for both the survivor and her family, which can begin to set the stage for developing maladaptive coping and communication skills [221].

Making decisions about cancer treatment is especially difficult as several treatment modalities exist, each with associated risks and benefits. The decision-making process is highly stressful, as patients are asked to consider an enormous amount of information, learn a new language, and make life-changing decisions. In addition, survivors often are faced with an inefficient health care system which further compromises survivors' abilities to make decisions, as well as to understand and weigh their health care providers' treatment recommendations [221,222].

Merely providing the information in the diagnostic stage is insufficient because survivors are reacting emotionally to the information and may not be able to fully process what they hear or read [5,221].

> "My first reaction was to think that I was going to die. I really didn't understand what the doctor was saying to me."

Research has shown that poor understanding and communication of information between patient and health care providers creates a barrier to well-being and increases distress [74,212,221,223-225]. According to the literature, interventions that favorably influence psychological and social functioning through enhanced coping skills need to be implemented as models for use as best practice [2,3,17,20,223,226,227].

> "I remember when the doctor was giving me this information, I'm listening. I'm listening. It's a lot of information. And then after he's finished – I don't know – I just couldn't remember stuff and I asked questions, but he replied … "I already told you that. You weren't listening." It is hard to take in all the information at one time."

A recent Institute of Medicine (IOM) report, *Cancer Care for the Whole Patient: Meeting Psychosocial Needs*, emphasizes the importance of quality services along the full spectrum of the cancer care continuum [10]. The continuum of breast cancer care is broadly conceptualized as prevention, early detection, diagnosis, disease management, supportive care, survival and survivorship. In large part, literature has focused more on prevention, early detection strategies and the time period between diagnosis and treatment rather than how needs change across the continuum.

> "When treatment finally ended, my husband was saying, "This is what you've worked toward all this time – to be free of the treatment." I said, "but I feel like I've been abandoned." I felt very alone. And my friends who were wonderfully supportive during when I was getting treatment now figured everything was OK with me. "This is wonderful. You're all done. This is terrific." Then it was like they'd call once a week instead of everyday and then maybe once a month or none at all."

Although numerous research efforts have been taken to address the various medical and psychosocial needs of survivors at a given point in their cancer experience, little research has been conducted on the trajectory of support needs for women from time of diagnosis to survivorship and remission [228-230]. Studies have shown, as indicated by Mullan (1985), that the cancer experience is best conceptualized as "seasons of survival" (diagnosis and treatment as the acute stage, remission as the extended stage, and permanent and end-of-life stage) [231].

"I was not introduced to a social worker at first, but now that I am with a new oncologist I was referred to a social worker. She helps with all my concerns – my medical concerns, my financial concerns, my emotions and everything. I wish I had known about her earlier on when I was first diagnosed."

Different from an acute illness, the stressors associated with cancer do not abate after each stage. Existing literature on the changing needs of women at various stages in their illness trajectory provides evidence that supportive care is needed throughout the cancer experience and should no longer be limited to the diagnosis/treatment phase [232]. Supportive care models, to date, tend to pivot around crisis points such as diagnosis, treatment, and post-treatment phases rather than seeing the stressors associated with the illness as ongoing [228].

"You need someone there from the beginning. It would be great if the social worker was there with you from the beginning and stayed with you."

There is a growing body of literature focusing on survivorship and the unmet needs of women re-entering their lives after cancer treatment. Recent studies and literature support Mullan's earlier assertions in 1985 that once treatment is over survivors are faced with a host of challenges ranging from physical limitations, social and economic concerns, fear of cancer reoccurrence and distress associated with the transition from patient to survivor [228,232,233]. In *Cancer Care for the Whole Patient: Meeting Psychosocial Needs* [234], an emphasis is made on framing the needs of these women within a whole person care context. Previously, researchers and practitioners have explored these women's needs with regard to managing their physical and psychological well-being at a given point in their cancer experience. In considering the whole-person care approach, practitioners must broaden their focus to include ongoing communications and psychosocial interventions as women transition from one stage to another.

"Later is the worst part of treatment. It sounds crazy, but there was something comforting about being in treatment. At least I was around the doctors and nurses. When treatment finished I felt very alone. This was the hardest part for me. Everyone expected me to be back to normal, but I didn't even know what normal was anymore."

ASSESSING FOR DISTRESS

It can be difficult to tell if survivors are experiencing "normal" distress or if their distress is "more serious." It is essential for oncology social work to assess for distress and measure distress on an ongoing basis. The American Cancer Society and the National Coalition for Cancer Survivorship developed a simple distress scale based on the pain scales often found in physicians' offices. The pain scales usually ask, "How is your pain right now on a scale from 0 – 10?" A score of 5 or above generally flags the treatment team of a problem with pain for this patient [235,236]. This scale assesses distress on the same 10-point scale in the following areas:

1. Practical Problems (e.g., housing, insurance/financial, work/school, transportation, childcare)
2. Family Problems (e.g., dealing with partners, dealing with children)
3. Emotional Problems (e.g., worry, fears, sadness, depression, nervousness, loss of interest in usual activities)
4. Spiritual/Religious Concerns
5. Physical Problems (e.g., pain, nausea, fatigue, sleep, getting around, bathing/dressing, breathing, mouth sores, eating, indigestion, constipation, diarrhea, changes in urination, fevers, skin, nose dry, tingling, swelling, sexual, appearance, memory/concentration).

This scale is particularly helpful for social workers because it is simple to use in the clinical setting, simple to score, and targets the areas generally viewed as social worker's domain [237]. This tool is currently being used routinely in screening distress in some larger cancer treatment centers [238].

Distress is an important part of the cancer experience, yet often overlooked by the treatment team. Social workers need to take a leading role in assessing distress in women with cancer. Screening tools, such as The Distress Scale, make screening for distress easy and efficient in the clinical setting. It is recommended that this tool become a routine part of the patient assessment.

Chapter 9

SPIRITUALITY

"Spirituality is a very personal, individual, daily… how you are living to get through the day, where you draw your strength from."

As mentioned in the previous chapter, a woman's distress following a cancer diagnosis may be not only emotional or psychological, but also spiritual as well. Although many women report using spirituality as a coping mechanism to give them strength along their cancer journey, not all women consider the spiritual dimension of their experience in a positive light. Unfulfilled spiritual needs can exacerbate feelings of emotional and psychological distress, and may even impact the ultimate outcome of a woman's cancer treatment [239].

The terms 'spirituality' and 'religion' are often used interchangeably in the quantitative literature, but female cancer survivors in qualitative studies define them as two separate and distinct concepts. Religion tends to be viewed as organized and institutional, with one's relationship to God being guided by a group of commonly agreed upon principles within the particular religious community. One clear advantage to studying spirituality through the lens of religion is that religion is more easily quantifiable; researchers can use church attendance or the number of times a person prays as a measure of their religiosity [240]. While religion is thus defined by one's involvement in an external church community, spirituality is considered to be much more internal and unique to the individual. This broader definition allows more freedom for a woman to connect with a spiritual aspect of herself, but is also considerably more difficult to quantify and measure for the purposes of scientific study [240,241].

"So, as far as spirituality…… yes, there was a great source of strength, but I can't take the philosophy of "oh well, whatever God wants – yeah – here we go." That's why I'm saying it's strength and not acceptance for me."

A woman with existing religious beliefs and practices at the time of her cancer diagnosis may find her beliefs challenged. She may be angry at God for her illness or question God's existence at all.

"I often wonder why God let this happen to me. I did everything right … church, community, pray … but it did no good. I question God altogether."

After the initial shock of the diagnosis has worn off, however, many women return to their religious beliefs and call on them as a source of strength [242]. They may turn to God for help in understanding the lessons of their cancer journey, or be more aware of and express gratitude for the blessings God has bestowed in their lives [239]. The church and religious community can also be a source of support for a cancer patient's practical needs, such as transportation, child care, and meals. The sense of belonging that comes with such outward displays of support from members of a church can positively impact the outlook of a woman with cancer [243].

> "I would have never made it through this without my church family. They were there for me when I needed support."

A woman may find that a change in her religious perspective following a cancer diagnosis does not easily conform to the beliefs that she held about God prior to her diagnosis. In this situation, she is faced with the challenge of reframing the realities of her diagnosis to fit with her existing religious beliefs, or revising her belief system to better match her new perspective [244]. For many women, this challenge requires them to look beyond their traditional religious beliefs to explore other sources of strength, and to blend these new ideas into a broader spiritual perspective [239]. In this way, women develop their own unique spiritual outlook to serve as a coping mechanism through their diagnosis and treatment.

> "I've got a lot of faith but it's just different – till it happens to you, you could just never fathom what women go through."

Although levels of religious belief and participation vary widely across studies (depending on the geographic location, racial and ethnic composition of the sample, and variables used to measure religion), most women report spirituality playing a significant role in their everyday lives.

> "When I was diagnosed, my faith in God helped me stay strong."

Some women do equate their religious beliefs with spirituality, while others subscribe to a more general higher power that is present and helps guide their lives [245]. For these women, spirituality is not attached to a deity or even a specific being, but rather the existence of a deeper reality that brings meaning to their lives. Many women do not feel allegiance to a particular church or denomination but nonetheless feel a deep connection to their spiritual selves [239]. As previously discussed, spirituality tends to be individualized; unique to what brings meaning to the life of each person. Some women find spiritual connections externally, in their relationships with friends and family or in their daily work. Other women turn inward for spirituality, finding personal meaning in nature, meditation, arts, or music [241]. Still others find that keeping a journal or traveling to locations that they find particularly peaceful help them feel connected to their spiritual selves [157,246]. In facing a cancer diagnosis, a woman may become more aware of her spiritual beliefs which have always existed but which she never knew were there [239].

There is general consensus in the literature that a significant majority of cancer survivors are able to find benefits in their cancer experience, including improved relationships with family and friends, a greater appreciation of living each day, and a reevaluation of priorities to value what is truly important [243]. Studies have shown that women who report having more meaning in their life after a cancer diagnosis also report less spiritual distress, although the direction of this relationship is uncertain. In other words, while these two concepts are definitively associated, it is unclear whether having meaning in one's life subsequently reduces the spiritual distress one experiences, or if initial lower levels of spiritual distress allow a woman to more easily identify meaning in her life and her cancer diagnosis [244]. Regardless of the causal ordering of this relationship, spiritual involvement has been shown to have positive psychological effects, including lower levels of depression and anxiety and higher self-reported levels of well-being and quality of life [239].

"I would sit and have long conversations with God. I've had lots of conversations with God."

Additionally, there is growing research to suggest that lower levels of spiritual distress can have positive effects on the physical health of a cancer survivor, including stronger immune functioning, better adjustment to the side effects of cancer treatment, lower blood pressure, lower self-reported levels of fatigue and pain, and prolonged survival [239,243,244].

"I don't worry about anything. I just talk to God about it and just go on because I know we all got to die sooner or later."

Despite the numerous psychological and physiological benefits offered by spiritual involvement, research also exists to suggest that the relationship between psychological adjustment, health outcomes, and spirituality is not always a positive one [240]. For example, several studies report that women feel a sense of helplessness and a loss of control over their own lives when they are diagnosed with cancer, regardless of whether or not they consider themselves to be a religious or spiritual person [239,241,244]. While some women find spiritual comfort in placing the outcome of their cancer journey in the hands of God or another higher power, others take this perspective to a different level by using it as an avoidant coping strategy. Giving the control of their cancer outcome to an external power allows these women to feel absolved of their own responsibilities after a cancer diagnosis. It also deprives them of the opportunity to be an active partner in making decisions about their treatment and seeking information about their cancer, activities that could be a source of empowerment when so many other things seem out of their control [244].

"I might not understand it, but this is God's path for me and he has the power to heal me at any time. This is God's will, and I pray to him for the answers. He gives me strength."

For women with a fatalistic view of their cancer diagnosis, participation in their treatment is seen as a senseless endeavor. Fatalism suggests that all events, both good and bad, are predestined by fate and that people, therefore, have no control over their destinies. The sense of powerlessness that accompanies this perspective resigns people to develop a passive attitude toward life's events. A fatalistic attitude can create significant conflict in determining the course of cancer treatment, as women may feel that the emotional and physical toll of treatment are useless since the outcome of their cancer has been predetermined by fate [244].

"Religion is completely different in my personal life for me than my relationship with God, which is a spirit felt thing. You know you can go to church and not see a spiritual person at all. Religion is like 'are you Baptist,' 'are you Catholic?' something like that. But I have a personal relationship with Jesus Christ and that's what gets me through. I've searched for why, why, why, and I cried. And what I have come to face with is that there's not an answer to why. Why me? I'm going to die, but I believe firmly that at any moment Christ has complete power and will to heal me."

This perspective may be most evident in populations where religious belief is an especially significant part of daily life, such as African American, Hispanic, or other non-Caucasian ethnic women or women living in rural communities [140,247,248]. This fact is problematic as these are the same populations that tend to be diagnosed with later stages of cancer and have shorter life expectancies after diagnosis. Fatalistic views of cancer and treatment are reinforced when women see neighbors, friends, or family members lose their battle with cancer despite undergoing treatment, even though the outcome has more to do with late stage of diagnosis and limited availability of treatment resources, rather than fate or destiny.

"I don't have a religious thing as far as that goes. I am strictly – up to me, up to the medical field, and I'm going to fight, and I'm going to depend on them, and I'm going to listen to them, and I'm going to do what they say. That's my way of getting through. I have had religion in the past … I have had things happen where religion failed me completely. I haven't got a whole lot to say for having that whole religious thing on my side."

A woman's cancer experience can be influenced not only by her own religious and spiritual beliefs, but also by those of her friends, family, and community. Being confronted with judgmental religious views can cause further spiritual distress for a cancer patient, who may question how her own beliefs align with those around her. She may even begin to consider the validity of these judgments, wondering if she indeed did bring the cancer upon herself.

"People question why you get the cancer. My religious neighbor suggested that God gave me the cancer because I had not been faithful enough."

Many female cancer patients experiencing spiritual distress do not have the opportunity to share their feelings with others, often out of a fear of being judged as spiritually weak [249,250].

"I never felt like I was punished. A lot of people feel like they're being punished, but I never felt like I was being punished. And to this day I think that the Lord had a plan for me."

The spirituality of close family and caregivers also influences the spiritual experience of a woman with cancer. Research has shown that, even if a woman reports a strong sense of personal spirituality, her spouse and children often report significantly lower levels of belief. Women who rely on their faith or spirituality as a coping mechanism will often discover that their beliefs are not shared or nurtured by their closest family members, making them feel that they are facing that part of the cancer journey alone [245].

"My husband and kids don't have faith in the power of God like I do. I pray every night and know that he will heal me."

Research has also shown that psychological distress is high in caregivers of women diagnosed with cancer when the caregiver has lower levels of spirituality. This association is strongest in female caregivers of a first-degree relative with breast or ovarian cancer, presumably because it forces them to face not only their increased risk for developing these cancers, but also their own mortality and that of their relative with cancer [251]. Caregivers who are struggling with their own psychological and spiritual distress are unable to provide the spiritual nurturing needed by the female cancer patient. Many researchers agree that social support and close personal relationships are key factors to spiritual well-being by helping the cancer survivor stay connected to sources of meaning in life. It is important for a woman who has been diagnosed with cancer to have opportunities to develop and nurture relationships with others who can identify with her spirituality, especially if she is not receiving that spiritual support from family members [244].

Oncology social workers are in a unique position to encourage and nurture the spiritual nature of the female cancer survivor. While research has shown that spirituality can have a positive impact on health outcomes for cancer patients, this should not be the primary reason for including spirituality in treatment; instead, social workers and physicians should address issues of spirituality out of respect for the survivor as a whole person rather than just a diagnosis [241,252,253]. As previously discussed, physicians and other medical professionals are generally untrained to explore issues of spirituality with their patients. Even those who are aware of the possibility of unmet spiritual needs in their patients often feel that asking about these needs is outside the scope of their work. Research has shown, however, that the majority of cancer patients feel it is appropriate for members of their treatment team, including social workers, to inquire about their spiritual needs [252]. Cancer patients with unmet spiritual or existential needs report a lower satisfaction with the care provided by their treatment team and perceive that care to be of lower quality. Oncology social workers can play a key role in influencing the quality of care for female cancer survivors by validating the existence of their spirituality and helping them to understand how these beliefs influence their cancer experience [253].

"My medical team never discussed my religion or spirituality with me. They never knew how much I depended on God to get me through this."

As a part of the oncology treatment team, social workers have the important responsibility of identifying unmet spiritual needs and helping the cancer survivor identify personal and external resources to actively cope with this distress. Social workers should take caution, however, that their own spiritual beliefs do not overshadow those of the survivor. It is important to be supportive and non-judgmental, even if their beliefs are incongruent with those of the survivor [245]. Providing an open, nurturing, and understanding environment for women to voice their spiritual beliefs in light of their cancer diagnosis allows them to feel safe exploring all possible spiritual coping tools, particularly for those women whose family and friends have belief systems different from their own [245]. Encouraging female cancer patients to identify what is important to them and what brings meaning to their life in turn helps all members of the treatment team, including the survivor, make the best treatment decisions based on a holistic view of the survivor and her needs.

Chapter 10

PROVIDING PSYCHOSOCIAL CARE: EVIDENCE BASED INTERVENTIONS

"Some days I just didn't want to get out of bed, and I didn't care if I never woke up. Everyone says keep a positive attitude, but it is easier said than done."

ASSESSING FOR PSYCHOLOGICAL CONCERNS

Although the U.S. may be one of the leaders in treating the medical symptoms of cancer, we are lagging behind in the psychosocial care of these women and their families. Australia is leading the world in establishing evidence-based guidelines. Along with national guidelines for the management of early and advanced breast cancer, Australia's National Health and Medical Research Council (NHMRC) recently has endorsed and published clinical practice guidelines for the provision of psychosocial care [254]. These guidelines were developed to provide the entire treatment team with evidence-based recommendations toward which they can strive in order to ensure that all women diagnosed with breast cancer receive optimal psychosocial care throughout all phases of treatment.

According to the American Cancer Society, ongoing effective communication between a health care professional and the patient is a clinical and public health priority. The National Coalition of Cancer Survivorship and the American Psychosocial Oncology Society have endorsed the development of screening procedures to improve the detection and management of emotional distress in cancer patients [12,255]. These guidelines emphasize the need to conduct an initial screening for distress at the time of diagnosis and continue screening through survivorship. Literature supports the conclusion that cancer patients are empowered by effective and frequent communications with members of their medical team [256-258]. Despite clear evidence on the importance of communication and a working relationship among women with cancer, women continue to report frustration in understanding and discussing personal issues with their physicians [258,259]. More importantly, different communication styles may lead to disparities in patient outcome. By establishing an early and ongoing interpersonal relationship with their treatment team, women are more likely to have improved outcomes such as adaptive coping skills and quality of life than women lacking such a relationship [259].

Many women with cancer will need some degree of support in adjusting to their diagnosis and treatment, and a smaller proportion of women will develop more severe psychiatric problems.

"When I finished treatment, I became very depressed. I was afraid it would come back. They actually sent me to see a psychologist and my social worker helped me a lot too."

A diagnosis of cancer may act as the trigger for the development of severe psychiatric illness. Screening for psychological distress can be easily done at times of diagnosis and recurrences, and oncology social workers should play a key role in this assessment. All women with cancer should be informed that counseling is available for themselves and their families, if needed.

"My emotions are on a roller coaster … up and down based on tumor markers. I seem to live from day to day for a change in my tumor markers."

Family members and friends often struggle with the emotional changes in the cancer survivors and struggle with whether these changes are psychological or due to the medications. Family members often report that the treatments have made the survivor "crazy," and they struggle with how to cope with these emotional changes.

"I'm not sure if my wife is bi-polar or if the chemotherapy is just making her crazy. I hate to bring up the topic with her because she thinks I'm not being supportive."
"I know my daughter would normally not act so crazy like this. It must be the high doses of chemo. She is so angry and mean now. I don't know what to do with her anger. Why is she mad at me? We are all really worried about her."

The emotional impact of cancer does not always go away when treatment ends. Women often feel the emotional impact of this disease into long-term survivorship, which can be very difficult on family and friends.

"I just want her to go back to normal. I thought when treatment ended that things would be better, but she still seems to be on an emotional roller coaster. When will this end?"

Many women with cancer will not need any additional psychosocial support or counseling; however, all women and their families should be empowered with the knowledge that these services are available and beneficial. The social work profession is in a key position to educate women and other health care professionals on the importance of psychosocial care for women diagnosed with cancer. In order to screen for psychological concerns, oncology social workers should do the following:

Document High Risk Factors
- Identify and document any high risk characteristics of the woman (e.g. young age, poor social support, children under 21 years of age, economic adversity, past psychiatric problems, interpersonal problems, etc)
- Identify and document any high risk disease characteristics (e.g. increased side effects, lymphoedema, recurrence, etc.)

Ask about General Functioning
Use model questions, such as:

- "In addition to looking at the medical/surgical issues, I am interested in hearing how things are going more generally for you"
- "How have you been feeling emotionally?"
- "Could you tell me how your mood is?"
- "How are you handling the diagnosis and treatment?"

Ask about Specific Clinical Issues
Use model questions, such as:

- "Diagnosis and treatment for breast cancer is often stressful for the couple and members of the family. Can you tell me how things are at home? How are your partner and family handling it?"
- "Some women find that they get quite depressed during treatment. If that is the case, there are a number of treatments available. I was wondering if you could tell me how your mood has been?"
- "Although it is often hard to talk about, many women feel concerned about how they look and feel about themselves after surgery and treatment. Can you tell me how you feel about these things? Are these concerns related to your decision about treatment? Have you discussed any concerns with your partner?"
- "Some women have a lot of worries about cancer and the treatment for it. What kind of worries do you have? How are you dealing with these worries?"
- "Having cancer affects many aspects of women's lives. One of the things that often concerns women, but which they may find hard to talk about, is their sense of themselves as a woman, and their intimate relationships. Can you tell me if there are any things like that that are worrying you?"
- "One concern women often have, but which they may find had to talk about is their sex life and intimate relationships. Are you or your partner having any concerns about this area of your life?"

Refer for Counseling
- Tell the woman about the benefits of both individual and group counseling.
- Provide the woman with various referrals for either individual or group counseling.
- Ask the woman if she would like you to assist with arranging the appointment.
- Ask if the woman has any questions about counseling.
- Communicate concerns and treatment plan to other members of the treatment team.

*Modified from the National Breast Cancer Center in Sydney, Australia [254].

THE BENEFITS OF PSYCHOSOCIAL INTERVENTIONS FOR WOMEN WITH BREAST CANCER

Despite the fact that emotional distress and psychological well-being are clearly linked to issues of quality of life and quality cancer care, clinicians fail to recognize distress among cancer patients [200,260,261]. Most distress experienced by survivors is often underreported by service providers due to the lack of recognition and inquiry [260]. Survivors are often reluctant to discuss emotional or practical concerns with their health care providers, and clinicians generally do not probe into psychosocial areas of well-being [200]. As well, survivors are often unwilling to share their emotional feelings for fear of being labeled with a "psychological" problem or for fear of distracting members of the medical team away from the primary concern of curing the cancer [12,255].

"I only have 10 minutes with my doctor and I barely have enough time to talk about my treatment and physical problems. I can't waste that time telling him about how depressed I am! When you only have a short time, you have to prioritize."

"My doctor already thinks I'm crazy because I keep asking about 'alternative treatments' … if he knew I was depressed, he would really think I'm crazy."

Furthermore, medical professionals are often not trained or skilled at identifying or discussing psychosocial concerns [11-15]. They often assume that emotional distress and/or psychological problems are a normal part of the cancer experience. Depression and anxiety may occur in response to the impact of diagnosis and meaning of the cancer, but can also be triggered by neurological, metabolic, nutritional, and endocrine changes, as well as medication. There is also a tendency to underestimate or undertreat psychological problems once they have been identified [15,261,262].

"When you go to the doctor's office, he's not interested in your mental health. He is going to be paid for the procedure that he performs on your body."

For example, in a study of low-income women with breast or gynecological cancer, 12% of those identified with major depression were prescribed antidepressants and only 5% received psychological treatment [263]. Ryan and colleagues identified the following barriers clinicians face in addressing emotional concerns and distress with their patients: patient and clinician attitudes and beliefs, patient's potential low level of health literacy, presence of physical symptoms taking precedence, and clinicians' lack of knowledge about distress [264]. Social workers have the knowledge and skills to ensure that women with cancer are referred to appropriate services as well as the skills to facilitate both individual and group counseling.

"Last year, I checked myself into a psychiatric hospital. I couldn't deal with it period. I couldn't do it. I was having thoughts that I had never had before. I was having thoughts of doing something to myself and taking my two small children with me. I couldn't do it. Once I went to the hospital and I saw some of those people in the psych unit. I was like – I'm never coming back here again. Whatever I have to face, I just have to deal with it."

Randomized controlled trials have shown that women with cancer who were provided with an opportunity to explore feelings with a member of the treatment team or a counselor had less psychosocial distress than women not provided with this opportunity [212,227,265,266]. Over the last two decades, Ganz and colleagues have shown that ongoing assessments are beneficial to identify at-risk breast cancer patients as well as promote self-care that maximizes biopsychosocial functioning during and after the acute phases of cancer treatment [4,211,213,232,267-272].

Cumulative evidence now clearly demonstrates that cancer patients benefit from psychosocial interventions [221]. A meta-analysis of 116 intervention studies showed that cancer patients receiving psychoeducational or psychosocial interventions had significantly lower rates of anxiety, depression, mood disturbances, nausea, vomiting and pain and significantly greater knowledge about disease and treatment relative to no-intervention controls [265]. Similarly, a meta-analysis of 37 published, controlled studies that investigated the effectiveness of psychosocial interventions on quality of life in adult cancer patients support the usefulness of psychosocial interventions for improving quality of life in adult cancer patients [273].

There is less evidence to indicate the best model of therapy for particular clinical settings, but many therapies have much in common [221]. For example, evidence from meta-analyses of randomized controlled trials indicates the efficacy of both supportive and cognitive-behavioral therapies in the treatment of depressive disorders in women with cancer [265], and the efficacy of both individual and group therapies [221]. It may be that the features of therapy common to all psychological interventions such as an empathic manner, listening, affirmation, reassurance, and support generate the observed outcome. Another meta-analysis found that the most important moderating variable in improving quality of life outcomes for cancer patients was duration of psychosocial intervention, with durations of more than 12 weeks being significantly more effective than interventions of shorter duration [273].

Based on a number of randomized control trials and two meta-analyses, there is evidence for a range of psychosocial interventions in all stages of cancer [221]. Psychosocial interventions may include cognitive-behavioral therapy, psychotherapy, psychoeducational therapy, group therapy, and family and/or couple therapy. Furthermore, interventions that target a holistic approach integrating mind body interventions (e.g., yoga, relaxation, stress management, etc.) have shown promise in providing long-term results in improving quality of life of women survivors [274].

In addition, literature shows telephone-based case management is highly effective in monitoring and addressing rehabilitation needs of cancer patients [268,275-278]. Telephone monitoring, as a form of case management, has long been used as a cost-effective social work intervention [279,280] with a primary focus on improving functional status and quality of life. Frequency in monitoring allows the social worker and the survivor to establish a long-term relationship designed to include direct provisions of counseling in the form of reassurance, referral to community resources, patient advocacy, adaptive skills training and early intervention.

Telephone counseling is emerging as a promising alternative to traditional counseling methods with cancer survivors. Polinsky and colleagues used a telephone monitoring intervention to follow 69 newly diagnosed breast cancer survivors for a year [268]. Findings indicate that a breast cancer survivor's needs and concerns changed over the trajectory of their cancer experience. In the first three months, women were more likely to complain about low energy, followed by psychological concerns and side effects of treatments. As treatments subsided, women discussed an increase in anxiety and fears associated with recurrence. As survivorship extended, women became more concerned with non-cancer related physical health issues. Overall findings showed women receiving additional information 38% of the time, reassurance over 58% of the time, and referrals to community resources 4% of the time.

The advantages of using a telephone-based intervention included limited staff requirements, cost-effectiveness, non-intrusive and flexible intervention, patient convenience, elimination of missed or canceled appointments, use of existing community resources, periodic risk assessments, timely referrals, and most importantly a professional commitment to provide ongoing medical and psychosocial support throughout the cancer experience [268]. Telephone-based interventions are a promising model for meeting the needs of rural cancer survivors, who do not have access to traditional support services. In considering the whole-person care approach, social workers must broaden their focus to include ongoing communications and psychosocial interventions as women transition from one stage to another [10].

SUPPORT GROUPS

Psychosocial support groups and psychoeducational groups are increasingly being recognized as effective cancer interventions in reducing psychological distress, and stress-related somatic complaints by enhancing basic coping skills [209,212,281]. Participants of cancer support groups have identified various benefits resulting from such groups including, mutuality and cohesion [282]; a sense of belonging and empathy; demystifying the unknown by providing educational information [283]; and creating a sense of community in place of isolation [281]. Psychosocial support groups have been found to significantly improve psychosocial well-being and minimize distress associated with the cancer diagnosis and treatment [212,284], particularly if they offer avenues of education, the opportunity to share experiences, and enhance basic coping skills [273,285,286].

Psychoeducational groups are structured groups led by trained professionals that emphasize learning and developing new life skills within a group setting [283]. Psychoeducational groups emphasize raising clients' awareness and helping individuals make sound decisions concerning issues in their lives. Research suggests that professionally led psychoeducational interventions are more effective than peer discussions, and those with longer duration are more effective than short-term interventions [273,285].

Itzhaky and York's research implied that women seek internal organizational control and participatory processes that lead to empowerment more than men [23]. By enhancing women's abilities to ask questions about their disease and treatment by educating them on how to seek this information through psychoeducational groups, it is more likely that women will effectively advocate for themselves. Individuals living with cancer need to have a place to go where they feel connected to others, can express feelings about their illness, and share and gain information to increase coping and adaptation to life with cancer.

"I only felt like talking about it to people going through it. I couldn't talk to my family or friends or anybody else, just the other girls who had gone through it."

One way in which the psychosocial needs of cancer patients can be addressed is through peer support groups, which are often recommended to patients by health care professionals. Peer support groups provide a safe, nurturing environment for people with cancer to alleviate emotional distress associated with their illness and offer opportunities to connect with others experiencing similar events.

"You were asking again about what the group does – for me, it's a group – it's a social group. It's a group of caring and sharing for whatever your needs are. But it's also a way of connecting with other women with the same condition and understanding. Like we all sit here and we all of us had breast cancer, but we didn't all have the same kind. We didn't all have the same treatment. We don't have the same everything, so what it does for us, at times, it's a matter of just getting together and sharing. And then you develop – from this group we have developed friendships. And this is something else – it adds to your friendship. We don't sit there and mope over it and grind over 'I have it' – 'I have it but what do I do with it.' You know what I'm saying? You move on."

While many hospitals and oncology clinics offer on-site support groups, some cities have community-based cancer support organizations. These organizations are non-clinical settings that, in addition to offering support groups for people with cancer, offer recreational, spiritual, and social programs for these individuals as well as their family members. There are a plethora of community cancer support organizations and wellness organizations around the country. For example, Gilda's Club is a cancer support community, which was founded in 1995 following the death of comedian Gilda Radner [287]. It was Radner's wish that cancer support communities be established around the world where people with cancer and their loved ones did not feel alone and would be able to gain support from those experiencing the same things. This idea is consistent with research that has shown that when people want to talk about personal issues, they prefer to speak with individuals with similar problems, a principle which encompasses mutual-aid support communities like Gilda's Club [288]. Gilda's Clubs around the country offer a place for people with cancer of all ages, their family members, and their friends to gain emotional and social support.

"Gilda's is the best thing that could ever happen to people with cancer and their families. It is a blessing and very helpful…."

Gilda's Club offers all programs free of charge and thus is accessible to anyone touched by cancer. Each Gilda's Club location offers weekly support groups for people with cancer and for family members and friends. The groups are not closed and allow new members to start at any time. The support groups are not time-limited and ask participants for at least a 16-week commitment, but ultimately leave it up to the participant to decide when he or she wishes to terminate [287]. Bereavement groups are also available for those who have lost loved ones to cancer. In addition, Gilda's Club offers workshops, classes, lectures and networking groups which are centered on a particular topic. Examples of these offerings are yoga and tai chi classes, spirituality, art classes, relaxation and guided imagery, and lectures given by health care professionals. Gilda's Club also offers members an opportunity to socialize with each other through monthly potluck dinners, movie nights, music concerts, and seasonal parties. One study on the experiences of survivors at Gilda's Club revealed that survivors were most interested in those groups which focused on skills to cope with their illness (e.g., relaxation, healthy cooking, self-hypnosis, etc.) [289].

There is a growing trend in online support services. Online support groups and communities are now offering many of the same features of traditional face-to-face support groups. Studies have found that survivors used online support groups to discuss their medical conditions, share personal concerns, discuss coping strategies, and offer support to each other [290-292]. One study found that women with cancer are more likely to provide support in online groups, whereas men are more likely to provide information [293]. Although online support groups are a growing trend for cancer survivors, the research in this area is only beginning to emerge and lacks proper testing of its effectiveness [290]. Most of the online support groups are peer led, and more research is needed on professional led online support groups. This model has great promise in the future, especially for survivors who are too sick to attend traditional support groups, work full-time, have limited access to transportation, or live in rural areas. However, many women will not be able have access to this type of support due to lack of internet access and/or knowledge of how to use computers. Oncology social workers should assess if this type of support might be helpful for the survivor and her family and provide appropriate referrals, as needed.

Survivors are often faced with an inefficient health care system which further compromises survivors' abilities to make decisions as well as understand and weigh their health care providers' recommendations [221,222]. Merely providing the information in the diagnostic stage is insufficient, because survivors are reacting emotionally to the information and may not fully process what they hear or read [5,221]. Research has shown that poor understanding and communication of information between patient and health care providers creates a barrier to well-being and increases distress [3,221,223].

Although many gaps remain in the knowledge base of psychosocial interventions, evidence suggests that interventions are more effective when they are explicitly designed to enhance personal capacities, such as coping skills, relaxation, goal setting, and problem solving [214]. Skills development and improving coping skills are basic social work tenets of consumer empowerment, which facilitates a broader concept of self-advocacy. While some women will be more comfortable with the privacy of individual counseling, other women will benefit from group counseling where they can gain from sharing the commonality of their experience [221].

The evidence supporting the provision of psychosocial care to women with cancer is clear. The challenge for the social work professional now is to ensure that women are able to access appropriate help when needed.

Chapter 11

IMPACT ON FAMILY AND FRIENDS

"One thing is for sure, for better or worse …. I'm not the same person as I was before I went through this diagnosis and treatment. I don't think I can ever go back to being that same person."

As illustrated, a cancer diagnosis affects a woman in a deeply personal and complex way, in part because of its extensive impact on her family and friends. Women are often changed forever by a cancer diagnosis, and this change requires a shift from everyone around her. The change reported by women is often positive, leading women to be more self-aware.

"I am not the same woman I was before I was diagnosed with cancer. I am stronger now, I fight harder, and I look at life differently. It is sometimes difficult for my family to understand how this experience changed me forever."

The extent to which a woman has support and feels supported has been identified as an important factor in women's adjustment to cancer. Women with poor support are more likely to experience the additional burden of psychological difficulties. Good support from family and friends is a protective factor, and lack of support may be associated with a poorer emotional adjustment [294,295].

"My husband always said "She's fine", he didn't understand I just wanted to cry."

A survivor's personal support structures should be reviewed to identify key support people, and the treatment team should build strong links with the patient's key support people. One possible way to achieve this link is for the social worker to ask the woman who her primary support people are, then advocate to include these key support people in consultations and decision-making.

"You do kind of figure out after a while who you can go to for different kinds of support. I know if you need somebody where you can be brutally honest with them and tell them the most negative things you have to say, you kind of know – I know – I've got one friend in particular that I can say anything to her no matter how negative it may sound –doom and gloom. If I want to have a pity party for a few minutes, she's not going to deny me that. But then you have other friends – they're called working bees – if you need something in particular you know that's who you go to. If you want somebody to say, 'Honey, everything's going to be okay' you can go to your daddy or your husband and they'll go, 'Well honey, you're going to live forever.' ... If I wanted somebody to give me some TLC you know not to go to your husband. If you want some TLC you might go to one of your friends at church or something.'

It is important to note that unwanted support may increase rather than decrease psychological distress in women with cancer. A spouse or partner is not always the key support person of the patient, and may even be the source of stress rather than support.

"When I found out I was going to have to have breast surgery, my doctor told me to go home and discuss it with my husband. But I told my doctor, "Doctor, I love my husband. He loves me. But, this MY body! I have to make the decision about my own body." My husband was very upset and angry that I had my breast removed and he cried. He didn't think I should have removed my breast, but it is not his body."

While social support can be provided by family and friends, in at least some cases, women may be reluctant to share their feelings with partners or families.

"I just keep things to myself, some things just upset my family if they know."

"The first time I didn't tell anyone other than my husband. I couldn't deal with everybody else."

Additionally, family members themselves may have high rates of psychological morbidity and need external support themselves [75,221,296-300]. The importance of support for women with cancer is clearly documented in the literature; however, the extent to which women's and their families' supportive needs are being met in routine care following a diagnosis of cancer remains unclear. Data from a population based survey of Australian women with breast cancer found that women under 50 years of age were more likely than older women to express a need for a greater number of support services during and after treatment, including additional support for their families [301].

"I had to take care of my husband. He was falling apart and he had nobody but me to help him. I was sick and taking care of him too."

Inevitably relationships will change when one partner or family member gets sick. The crisis of a serious illness can bring a couple or family closer or it can drive them apart if not properly addressed. Cancer is a chronic disease so the demands of this disease continue long past the acute treatment phase. The usual dance of dependence, independence, and interdependence encounters a shift. The partner of a cancer patient often moves into a caregiver role. The National Cancer Institute defines a "caregiver" as a family member or friend who helps a loved one manage cancer treatment. This can range from day-to-day activities to doctor visits to medical care options [302].

"It's actually the family who suffers because there is nobody to help them through the process. I have my medical team, but my family had no one."

Being a caregiver is not always easy since the emotional, mental, and physical demands are so high. This new role can be especially difficult for men, who have not been socialized into this role. Caregivers are often called upon to negotiate a difficult health system, advocate for services, negotiate with insurance companies, or manage the household and children [303]. Many are doing all of this and more.

> "I think there should be a plan, just like there are therapies for domestic abuse families and therapies for abused children, there should be therapy that would teach the family what a person with cancer is like and how they feel."

There is no question that a relationship will be tested throughout this period. It should be noted, however, that it is atypical for cancer to be the cause of divorce or separation. Most relationships that are secure before a cancer diagnosis remain intact after surgery and treatment [304].

Trust, honesty, and communication are necessary for maintaining satisfying intimate relationships [305], and studies report that people have more likelihood of thriving emotionally in a crisis, like cancer, if they have strong relationship ties [306]. How cancer patients and families cope with the experience of cancer can directly influence perceived levels of hope and suffering [307]. Because the emotional, physical, and relational challenges confronting a woman diagnosed with cancer and her family vary across the cancer continuum, it is helpful to discuss potential changes and coping strategies for the cancer patient's partner, children, and other family members and friends in the general stages of diagnosis, treatment, and survival [304].

How Does a Cancer Diagnosis Affect Partners?

After learning of a cancer diagnosis, the partner of the cancer patient may encounter a range of conflicting emotions. Oftentimes, news of a diagnosis comes so quickly that there is not a great deal of time to take and process it. A knee-jerk need to collect information, resolve problems, and be protective can inundate the partner and he/she may not know where to begin. For some, the need for information may help regulate their emotional balance. It might be helpful to suggest that the partner begin keeping a journal to write down the date and time of every doctor's visit, in addition to every procedure suggested or performed. It might also be helpful to suggest that the partner request to tape-record consultations and to obtain printed information regarding treatment options.

> "We have a very close relationship – without her I am nothing. The doctor said that it was very rare for a husband to accompany his wife to her visits. I go to all of them with her."

There is a high likelihood that partners will be anxious about the future and potential loss of his/her loved one. He/she also may be confronted by his/her own mortality for the first time in his/her life. Common reactions include fear, anger, denial and a sense of betrayal. Another typical feeling experienced by partners is self-inflicted guilt. They may personally experience intense emotional turmoil yet know their significant other is already burdened with the news of her cancer diagnosis. Therefore, the partner's feelings may go unaddressed.

Research demonstrates that male caregivers may be more comfortable sharing their feelings in a men-only forum or group [308].

While the woman living with cancer may be trying to renegotiate the transition from supporter to supported, the healthy partner assumes it is his/her responsibility to be the dominant, stable one in the relationship so as not to interfere with his partner's stress [304].

> One patient stated: My husband didn't understand. He was like – somebody at work would say," Oh, is she okay?" and he goes, "Yeah, she's fine" and so he'll come home, "Oh, so and so wanted to know if you're okay, and you're okay aren't you?" and I'm like (makes throwing up sounds). He angered me quite a bit because he didn't want me to feel bad. He was always telling everybody I was fine, but all I wanted to do was cry. And a couple of times I cried, and he was angry at me for crying, and he would say, "You're fine. Dr. X said you're going to be just fine," and I'm like, "but I still just want to cry."

The partner needs to be given permission to acknowledge their own needs and fears. The focus is generally on the patient, while the partners are often left without the skills needed to help themselves or their partner.

> "My husband could not handle me being sick and this disrupting his life and his schedule. I remember being in the chemotherapy room all strapped up and my husband just yelling and cussing at me. He was saying terrible things to me! The nurse walked by and just looked at me. I was so embarrassed. He never could handle my disease. He left me with two young children and advanced breast cancer."

There are many options for partners, including individual counseling, support groups for partners, or finding a support person for the partner to talk with [303]. For some people, a cancer crisis brings out their strengths and good qualities; for others, it amplifies their weaknesses and negative qualities. It is also difficult for partners and families to deal with the chronic impact of a cancer diagnosis. They often expect the survivor to be back to "normal" once acute treatment is complete. One of the challenges for the partner and the couple is to find a "new normal" and come to terms with the long-term effects of cancer and its treatments.

> "I just miss the woman I married. She has changed so much. I don't know where to go from here."

It is important to assess the extent to which the survivor would like her partner to be involved in decision making and treatment planning. Some women prefer their partners to be very involved in treatment decisions; however, others may feel that it is their body and their decision to make alone.

> "My husband found all this information on the internet and always disagreed with my doctors. He got angry at me for listening to my doctors. I know he was trying to help me, but it made me very frustrated and angry at him."

Encouraging communication between survivors and partners should be priority since silence can be interpreted as a lack of interest. Couple therapy among women with cancer has been shown to reduce emotional discomfort in both partners, increase communication, reduce depression in the woman, and increase sexual satisfaction for both partners [309,310].

"My husband just walked away. He couldn't handle a sick wife so he left. No one ever talked to us about counseling. If I had not been so sick, I probably would have fought harder to make our marriage work, but I didn't have the energy."

Despite its connection to quality of life, sexuality is often overlooked as an important issue in the health care setting [305]. Information about the impact of cancer and cancer treatment is often insufficient and not presented at appropriate times [311]. A woman and her partner's sexuality should be considered throughout all phases of the cancer experience. Many of the side effects of cancer treatment—pain, fatigue, nausea, skin irritation, headaches, and hormone changes--can impact a person's self-esteem and sexuality. For those living with cancer and taking medication for depression and anxiety treatment, this holds especially true. Physically, radiation therapy can cause swelling and irritation in the breast or arm. Lovemaking may not be a top priority for her at this time. Cancer treatment can induce early menopause in some women, which may mean hot flashes, vaginal dryness and thinning of vaginal walls. These menopausal symptoms can cause painful intercourse and postcoital bleeding [304]. Sexuality is not restricted to the act of sex. It also refers to the unique attributes manifest in a person and expressed through the body, mind, and soul.

Physicians often avoid asking questions about sexuality and body image. The oncology social worker or a member of the treatment team should ask model questions, such as,

"Having cancer affects many aspects of women's lives. One of the things that often concerns women, but which they may find hard to talk about, is their sense of themselves as a woman, and their intimate relationships. Can you tell me if there are any things like that that are worrying you?"

"One concern women often have, but which they may find hard to talk about is their sex life and intimate relationships. Are you or your partner having any concerns about this area of your life?"

Survivors and their partners often feel uncomfortable discussing these types of issues with their doctor, but may feel more comfortable talking with the oncology social worker. To help foster sexual intimacy and to combat disagreements stemming from misunderstandings, women and their partners should be encouraged to discuss their sexual expectations openly. Addressing sexual expectations can include fears, frequency, preferred positions, and times of the day when the survivor feels best [304].

The internet is also becoming an important tool in dealing with sexuality issues associated with the cancer experience. For example, as part of a larger "ask the experts" web service, there is now a sexual health awareness column which provides a safe venue to obtain information on how to deal with changes in sexual functioning due to cancer and cancer treatment [311].

Treatments following surgery like chemotherapy and radiation therapy have a range of physical side effects spilling over into emotional side effects, both of which need care. Every chemotherapy agent has temporary side effects which can last hours or days. Some women have very few side effects while others experience a wide range of effects. Physical side effects can include fatigue, nausea, dry skin, cracked nails, mouth sores, and menopausal symptoms such as hot flashes, vaginal dryness, and the end of menstruation altogether. It is important to discuss with partners and family members that the side effects of cancer may continue during and after the treatment process. Survivors and their family members are often prepared for the acute stage of cancer, but they are not prepared for the chronic effects of cancer treatment.

> "Everyone wants you to get back to 'normal' after the surgery and treatment, but no one understands the constant pain. They just think you are all better and need to get on with life, but I'm still in pain."

Partners and family members often experience emotional distress as a result of the cancer diagnosis; however, the focus is generally on caring for the survivor as opposed to caring for loved ones. The emotional strain of renegotiating roles within the relationship can also be burdensome. It is difficult for them to be supportive while also coping with their own emotions. Partners and family members often lack the skills and resources to deal with their own emotions, or they feel guilty about their own negative feelings about what has happened to their lives. The unmet psychosocial needs of partners continue to affect partners into long-term survivorship [296,312].

Oncology social workers need to address the emotional concerns of family members and provide an opportunity for them to share their fears, negative thoughts, and emotions. It is important to normalize family members' experiences and connect them with resources to deal with their own issues. A diagnosis of cancer is often a life changing experience for women, and partners and family members need time and their own safe space to deal with these changes. They often think they have to be "strong" for the cancer survivor, which results in them not dealing with their own emotions. It is important for the oncology social worker to ask partners and family members how they are doing. Many organizations provide support groups or services for loved ones of cancer survivors. It is important to refer all those affected by cancer to resources that can address their own struggles and meet their needs.

HOW DOES MOM'S CANCER AFFECT KIDS?

A cancer diagnosis that comes at time when a woman is raising children brings with it multiple worries. When she first receives her diagnosis, a woman may experience anxiety over how to discuss her illness with her children, questioning the level of disclosure she should provide to them.

> "I didn't think so much about me when I was diagnosed. I was more worried about my children. I couldn't just fall apart. I had to be strong for them."

Some women find that there is a limited amount of information available to them about how to approach the difficult task of communicating news of illness to their children [78]. Age is an important factor in how children will react to the news of their mom having cancer. Explaining a breast cancer diagnosis can be especially difficult when the woman's children are younger.

"I have a 15 year old and a 10 year old and all I could think about was who is going to take care of them if I die? I have no one to look after my kids."

As treatment progresses, it is likely that children will have questions about the changes they perceive in their mother's energy level and physical appearance, such as hair loss as result of chemotherapy. Children will want to know how their own lives will change during the treatment process. They will also wonder if their mother will die. Mothers may experience anxiety over the appropriate way in which to respond when confronted with these difficult questions, wondering how honest she should be about how she feels and her prognosis [313]. It is recommended to consult a social worker, school counselor, or other parents who have gone through a similar situation [314].

"My kids were very worried about me. I took them to the doctor with me and I let him talk to them and explain to them."

As a woman attempts to cope with the roller coaster of emotions she finds herself on after she has found out she has cancer, it is likely she will also have concerns about the emotional wellbeing of her family as they too adjust to a cancer diagnosis in the household.

"Having support for family is great if you can get family to participate in support groups or counseling. My husband needs support most but doesn't want to come in. Men are especially vulnerable. My kids are also very resistant to help. My teenage daughter felt angry, but didn't want to get help."

On the one hand, a woman may strive to maintain openness and honesty with her children. Yet simultaneously , she may feel the need to appear "strong" in front of her family, compelled to hide her emotions from her children in order to protect them from seeing the pain, fear, and uncertainty she is experiencing [78]. Concealing her emotions and pretending courage and positivity can be exhausting, and a woman's need to look after the emotional health of her children throughout her illness may come at the expense of her own emotional self-care. Because children often sense a parent's feelings, even as she tries to hide them, honest and age-appropriate discussions with children about their mother's cancer diagnosis are recommended [87,314,315]. As with cancer survivors, all children are unique in their response to the experience of their mother's cancer. It is important to allow children to express their emotions in their own way and in their own time.

"I've been in and out of treatment since my kids were babies, so all they have ever known is sick mom. I wish they could understand how sick I feel, but it is just normal to them. They have no idea that I'm going to die soon and I don't know how or when to tell them."

A cancer diagnosis changes the entire family system, and children, especially older children, often are burdened with additional challenges and responsibilities. It is normal for children to experience a range of emotional reactions and for these emotions to change over time. Initially, children are often very helpful and want to take care of their mom, but over time they can become frustrated with the inconvenience that cancer is causing in their own lives. They may also be embarrassed by having a sick mom and miss their old "normal" life before mom was sick.

"When I first got sick my kids were so sweet and wanted to help me, but eventually they became angry that I was sick for such a long time. It was really hard on them when I couldn't do the same stuff for them."

Oncology social workers should assess the needs of women with children and provide appropriate resources to help both the parents and the children. There are excellent resources for children, (e.g., Kids Konnected, American Cancer Society, Children's Treehouse Foundation, and Gilda's Club) that the oncology social worker can provide to the family. The social worker can also play an important role in meeting with the family and children to provide information, counseling, and support. Social workers need to continually monitor the needs of women with children because their needs and situation can change over time, especially as the disease progresses into the end-of-life phase.

"My kids are 13 and 15 and I know I'm going to die. I have to prepare them for the end phase. It is so hard."

Chapter 12

ADVOCACY AND CANCER

"I needed a champion for my cause, but I felt so unprepared. How do I battle with my insurance company, my work, and keep my sanity all at the same time?"

Advocacy is one of the founding principles of social work. The history of social work is rooted in social action efforts of early community group workers. Oncology social workers are often called upon to "advocate" on behalf of the survivor and their family, especially when working with medically underserved populations. Social workers often advocate for survivors in ways that the survivors are unable to advocate for themselves. For example, oncology social workers often advocate to ensure that needed services are provided to survivors and their families (e.g., calling insurance companies, talking with hospital staff about needs of the patients, liaising with community organization, and advocating for change in policies).

Because it is impossible to always be there to advocate on behalf of the survivor, oncology social workers also need to teach survivors how to advocate on their own behalf. Survivors can advocate for themselves on an individual level and on a community and political level.

INDIVIDUAL LEVEL

On the individual level, advocacy focuses on a competency-based model that emphasizes skill development and coping strategies as a way of preventing and managing the demands associated with the cancer experience within the domains of psychological and social functioning [2,5,80,316]. Skills development is a basic social work tenet of consumer empowerment which facilitates a broader concept of self-advocacy. Clark and Stovall suggested, "advocacy is the cornerstone of survivorship" [17]. Survivorship research has identified five interrelated skills that can improve health outcomes:

1. communication,
2. ability to seek needed information,
3. problem solving,
4. decision-making,
5. negotiation skills, and

6.   one's ability to stand up for their rights [2,5,17,20,223].

The concept of advocacy for cancer survivors began in the cancer peer support community and later was embraced by professionally led organizations [2,3,317]. Although many gaps remain in the knowledge base of psychosocial interventions, evidence suggests that interventions explicitly designed to enhance personal capacities, such as coping skills, goal setting, and problem solving produce larger effect sizes than do interventions lacking those components [214]. Oncology social workers routinely assess the patient's functioning within the areas of psychological, social, and spiritual well-being and provide appropriate support, resources, and referrals for services to enhance the skills needed to improve functioning within these domains. Most health care providers have little time for any patient-related care other than traditional medical care, and few health care providers devote their limited resources to patient advocacy [2]. Most physicians, nurses, and other key treatment team members have not had formal education or training on how to advocate for their patients or assist them in self-advocacy [2].

> "I was very lucky to have a husband who knew how to negotiate with insurance companies because they tried to rip us off and refuse to pay just about every bill. I don't know what other women do that don't have someone to help them get through the red-tape."

Quality cancer care necessitates a multidisciplinary team approach that allows survivors to access experts other than physicians before, during, and after treatment [3]. Oncology social workers are in a unique position to be a key member of the treatment team and play a fundamental role in assisting in the psychosocial care and advocacy role for cancer survivors [4,5,318].

In 1998, the Cancer Survival Toolbox was created through a unique collaboration among the National Coalition for Cancer Survivorship (NCCS), the Oncology Nursing Society (ONS), and the Association of Oncology Social Work (AOSW) with an unrestricted educational grant from Genentech, Inc. [319]. Through years of research and direct service, these leading oncology organizations recognized the need to teach cancer survivors how to seek out information, make the best possible decisions about their care, and interact effectively with their health care team, insurers and employers [5,318]. Such a need for skills development is the primary strategy that facilitates the empowerment process by:

1.   enhancing experience and competencies;
2.   enhancing group structure and capacity;
3.   removing social and environmental barriers; and
4.   enhancing environment support and resources [320].

These leading oncology organizations decided the best way to teach these skills was to develop self-learning tools that cancer survivors and their family members and friends can easily understand and use [319]. Since its release, over half a million Cancer Survival Toolbox tape sets and compact discs have been distributed across the country. In fall 2002, a website was launched to make the Toolbox easily accessible to on-line users [319]. In addition to individuals using the Toolbox, a facilitator's manual has been established to use the Toolbox in a psychoeducational setting [319]. Oncology social workers can use the

Toolbox individually with clients or in a psychoeducational group setting (www.canceradvocacy.org/toolbox).

Other resources for self-advocacy for women and their families are available from the NCCS including:

- *Self-Advocacy: A Cancer Survivor's Handbook*
Ellen Stovall and Terry Campbell

- *Teamwork: The Cancer Patient's Guide to Talking with Your Doctor*
Elizabeth J. Clark (available in English and Spanish)

- *What Cancer Survivors Need to Know about Health Insurance*
Kimberly J. Calder and Karen Pollitz (available in English and Spanish)

- *Working It Out: Your Employment Rights as a Cancer Survivor*
Barbara Hoffman (available in English and Spanish)

- *You Have a Right to Be Hopeful*
Elizabeth Clark (available in English and Spanish)

- *A Cancer Survivor's Almanac: Charting Your Journey*
Barbara Hoffman

COMMUNITY AND POLITICAL ADVOCACY

There is a growing trend in health care for consumers to have an active voice in all decisions related to their care [321,322]. Consumer advocates are needed to ensure that services received are as equitable, accessible, effective, and efficient as possible. Traditionally, patient advocacy has been done by health care providers as opposed to patients themselves [4,323]. However, the AIDS activist movement saw an increase in patients advocating on their own behalf for changes in the health care system, research, and policy. This trend of patient advocates has also developed within the area of cancer [324-326].

The most successful example of breast cancer advocacy has been in the U.S. In 1991, a small group of consumers in the U.S. formed the National Breast Cancer Coalition with a goal to eradicate breast cancer through action and advocacy [327,328]. Since that time, the coalition has increased federal funding for breast cancer research more than 600% -- from less than $90 million before the Coalition began to over $2.1 billion; created a nationwide, grassroots advocacy network that consists of more than 600 member organizations and 60,000 individuals; and brought about the development of an unprecedented multi-million dollar breast cancer research project within the Department of Defense that has attracted more than 29,000 research proposals [329]. In addition, they have successfully ensured a consumer voice at the peer review research table, policy level, and other areas where decisions about breast cancer are being made [329].

As demonstrated in Brussels in 1997 at the First International Conference on Breast Cancer Advocacy funded by the National Breast Cancer Coalition, breast cancer advocacy is beginning to emerge around the world. More than 250 delegates from 44 countries and six continents attended the conference to discuss their experiences in breast cancer advocacy as well as strategies to mobilize action worldwide [325,327]. This conference clearly demonstrated the status of breast cancer advocates as equal partners with health professionals, scientists, and policymakers in improving and changing the current state of breast cancer care [325].

In order for consumers to be effective in advocating for change, it is essential that they have the knowledge and skills necessary to communicate with scientists, researchers, and health care professionals. In response to this need, the National Breast Cancer Coalition pioneered the training of breast cancer advocates in what they called project LEAD (Leadership, Education and Advocacy Development) in 1995. Project LEAD uses scientists to instruct advocates on the basic biology of cancer, epidemiology, and leadership skills [330]. Similar training and educational programs are currently being developed and/or offered in Australia, Canada, and some Western European countries. These programs have been shown to produce a significant increase in participants' involvement in serving as a member of a board or committee, working on clinical trials recruitment issues, working on patient resources, and being involved in breast cancer advocacy groups after completing the training program [324].

The National Coalition for Cancer Survivorship (NCCS) is the oldest survivor-led advocacy organization in the United States. Their goal is to advocate at the federal level for quality cancer care for all Americans and to empower cancer survivors to have a strong voice in their cancer care. In 2004, the NCCS launched a grassroots network, "Cancer Advocacy Now!", to give cancer survivors and their loved ones across the country a voice in advocating for quality cancer care. Participants are given the tools and training to learn how to apply their self-advocacy skills to effectively fight for quality cancer care at the national level. The program utilizes emails to alert participants to policy issues that require action from cancer survivors [319].

Another way that cancer survivors, family, and friends can become involved in community and political advocacy is through participating in community fundraising events and projects for cancer research and services. Many survivors and their family and friends become involved in fund raising activities and events, such as walkathons, charity runs, galas, golf tournaments, Bike for the Cure, Ride for the Cure, pink ribbon events, and numerous other cancer events. These activities often give survivors and their supporters an opportunity to become involved in making a difference in the lives of other women suffering from cancer. Participating in these types of events are a way to give something back, as well as an opportunity to network and gain support from others who have gone through similar experiences.

It is important to note that although these events can be very positive, they are often targeted at a specific diagnosis, usually breast cancer. Thus, women with other cancers may not have the same opportunities or feel excluded because they have another type of cancer.

"I have ovarian cancer, and my husband and I were standing to pick up our Race for the Cure packets next to the survivors' line. I had just completed my second round of chemo and was pretty skinny, balding,... and... well... cancer looking. My husband struck up a conversation with the three ladies working the survivors table. Since I obviously looked like a cancer patient, I was asked if I was a survivor... in response, the main lady at the table asked if I had breast cancer. Since I didn't, I told her that I had ovarian cancer, not breast cancer. Although she was very nice, she said something along the line of "why no honey, you're not a survivor but you are more than welcome to walk FOR survivors..." I was stunned that they did not consider me a "survivor".

Breast cancer is the most well-organized and most successful of the women's cancer group in terms of fundraising, public education, and research dollars. The focus on breast cancer often has negative implications for other lesser known cancer types. Unfortunately, cancer types are often fighting amongst themselves for limited research and treatment dollars as well as fighting amongst other disease groups (e.g., heart disease, HIV/AIDS, diabetes). More efforts similar to the National Coalition of Cancer Survivors should be encouraged so that all women feel a part of the fight to eradicate cancer as a larger group of cancer survivors.

Chapter 13

THE CHANGING WORLD OF TECHNOLOGY

"I don't even get on the internet because I just get overwhelmed and confused. There is so much information and everywhere I click it says something different."

One of the biggest changes in the health care world is access to information which is available to most people on the internet. This open access to information is a change for consumers as well as professionals. However, this new flood of information is often overwhelming for survivors as well as professionals, and can often have negative implications for survivors.

WEBSITES: WHERE TO TURN?

The Internet holds invaluable resources for survivors, families, friends, and professionals seeking information about cancer-related resources. But, as we all know, there can be problems finding them. The web is huge, so how can we trust the reliability of a particular source? Who is the sponsor or author of a site? These are crucial questions to consider when looking for trustworthy information.

According to a study done by the University of Texas in early 2008, five percent of breast cancer websites have mistakes, with those involving alternative or complementary medicine being more misleading [331]. Having access to reliable cancer information and literature is relatively easy using appropriate indexes, such as Cancerlit, Medline Plus, and Cancerlinks [332].

Below is a list of trustworthy resources that might be helpful to professionals, survivors, and their loved ones in looking for information and services on women's cancer:

- *National Comprehensive Cancer Network (NCCN)* (www.nccn.org) is an alliance of the world's leading cancer centers, and it is an authoritative source of information to help survivors, families, and professionals make informed decisions about care.
- *National Guideline Clearinghouse* (www.guideline.gov) is a comprehensive database of evidence-based clinical practice guidelines and related documents. Key components of this site include structured abstracts about the guideline and its development, links to full-text guidelines, an electronic forum, NGC-L, for exchanging information on clinical practice guidelines and an annotated

bibliography. There are also user-friendly links to other services and reports, as well as a glossary of terms commonly used in standardized abstracts.

- *American Society of Clinical Oncology (ASCO) guidelines* (www.asco.org) ASCO has gathered and synthesized data on breast cancer from a multitude of key sources, including the *Journal of Clinical Oncology* and other ASCO publications, the Virtual Meeting, and more.

- *European Society for Medical Oncology (ESMO)* (http://www.esmo.org/) is designed to improve the quality of information, disseminate knowledge in oncology to cancer patients and the public, educate and train persons involved in clinical cancer care and research, and facilitate equal access to optimal cancer care to all cancer patients.

- *CancerCare* (www.cancercare.org) is a website maintained by social workers to offer counseling, information, referrals, and educational services. The site also provides seminars and consultations for health care professionals involved with cancer patients.

- *Breast Cancer Online* (www.bco.org) aims to facilitate timely access to new trends and topical information in breast cancer for health care professionals. It includes articles, case studies, expert opinions, journal clubs, journal watch, visual library, and conference reports.

- *National Cancer Institute (NCI)* (www.cancer.gov) The NCI, established under the National Cancer Institute Act of 1937, is the Federal Government's principal agency for cancer research and training. The National Cancer Act of 1971 broadened the scope and responsibilities of the NCI and created the National Cancer Program. Over the years, legislative amendments have maintained the NCI authorities and responsibilities and added new information dissemination mandates as well as a requirement to assess the incorporation of state-of-the-art cancer treatments into clinical practice.

- *American Association for Cancer Research (AACR)* (www.aacr.org/main.asp) was founded in 1907 to assist researchers and physicians in communicating new findings in the field of cancer and related issues. In order to fulfill its mission, the AACR publishes six scientific journals, coordinates scientific conferences and educational workshops, offers grants for young researchers, and provides the public with educational programs.

- *American Cancer Society (ACS)* (www.cancer.org) The American Cancer Society's web site is an important extension of the Society's mission to provide lifesaving information to the public. The user-friendly site includes an interactive cancer resource center containing in-depth information on every major cancer type. Through the resource center, visitors can order American Cancer Society publications, gain access to recent news articles, and find additional on- and off-line resources. Other useful sections on the web site include a directory of medical resources, links to other sites organized by cancer type or topic, resources for media representatives, and information on the Society's research grants program, advocacy efforts, and special events.

- *American Breast Cancer Foundation* (www.abcf.org) provides women and men in financial need, regardless of age or race, access to breast cancer early diagnosis. The foundation also offers assistance to patients and their families, and supports research. They have provided direct financial assistance to tens of thousands of woman and men in need of diagnostic testing to rule out or confirm breast cancer and begin treatment.

- *American Institute for Cancer Research* (ACOR) (www.AICR) Since its founding in 1982, the American Institute for Cancer Research has grown into the nation's leading charity in the field of diet, physical activity and weight management as it relates to cancer prevention. AICR supports research into the role of diet and physical activity in the prevention and treatment of cancer. It also offers a wide range of cancer prevention education programs.

- *Association of Cancer Online Resources (ACOR)* (www.acor.org) is a unique collection of online communities designed to provide timely and accurate information in a supportive environment. The site includes links to mailing lists, support and resources, treatment options, and publications.

- *Gilda's Club Worldwide* (www.gildasclub.org) Gilda's Club is named in honor of Saturday Night Live comedian Gilda Radner, who died of ovarian cancer in 1989. Its mission is to develop strategies and lead activities that will enable its worldwide group of independent affiliates to become the premier emotional and social support community for people with cancer and their families and friends.

- *OncoLink* (www.oncolink.com) is the Internet cancer resource from the Abramson Cancer Center of the University of Pennsylvania. It provides information on types of cancer, treatment options, clinical trials and other resources. The unique feature of OncoLink is that it was the first multimedia cancer website on the Internet.

- *Cancer Information Service* (http://cis.nci.nih.gov/) is a service provided by the National Cancer Institute. Its main focus is providing updated information on scientific research for everyday people. The program does this by providing a toll-free telephone hotline for people with general questions about cancer, research, etc.

- *National Breast Cancer Coalition (NBCC)* (www.natlbcc.org) trains advocates to lobby at the national, state and local levels for public policies that impact breast cancer research, diagnosis and treatment. To achieve its mission of ending breast cancer, its focus is on three main goals, namely: research, access, and influence.

- *National Ovarian Cancer Coalition (NOCC)* (www.ovarian.org) provides survivors, families, and professionals with information about ovarian cancer and appropriate resources.

- *Women's Cancer Network (*www.wcn.org) provides women and their families with information and enables them to be their own health advocates. The Women's Cancer Network was developed by The Gynecologic Cancer Foundation.

- *National Coalition of Cancer Survivorship (NCCS)* (www.canceradvocacy.org) is the oldest survivor-led cancer advocacy organization in the country, advocating for quality cancer care for all Americans and empowering cancer survivors. NCCS believes in evidence-based advocacy for systemic changes at the federal level in how the nation researches, regulates, finances, and delivers quality cancer care.

RESOURCES FOR ONCOLOGY SOCIAL WORKERS

Information overload is frequently experienced by social workers and other professionals. New research emerges monthly in various peer-reviewed journals, reports, and on websites. Below is a sample list of peer-reviewed journals that might be useful for oncology social workers:

- Psycho-Oncology
- Palliative and Supportive Care
- The Journal of Psychosocial Oncology
- Journal of Cancer Survivorship: Research and Practice
- Supportive Care in Cancer
- The Journal of Supportive Oncology
- Cancer Nursing
- Journal of Social Work in End-of-Life and Palliative Care
- Acta Oncologica
- Health Psychology Review (HPR)
- European Journal of Oncology Nursing
- Seminars in Oncology Nursing
- Journal of Pediatric Oncology Nursing
- European Journal of Cancer Care
- Journal of Clinical Oncology
- Journal of Health Communication
- Annals of Behavioral Medicine
- Journal of Loss and Trauma: International Perspectives on Stress and Coping
- Journal of Cancer Pain and Symptom Palliation
- The Breast
- The Breast Journal
- Breast Cancer Research and Treatment
- Breast Cancer Research
- Clinical Breast Cancer

Many of the journals now have full-text articles available online, and oncology social workers often have access to these journals through their organizations or public libraries. Google Scholar is an excellent tool to search for academic based articles and reports.

The main challenges for oncology social workers is staying up-to-date with the latest information and synthesizing the enormous amount of literature on any given topic related to areas of specialization. With the new focus on evidence-based practice, oncology social workers are feeling increasing pressure to ensure that they are delivering 'evidence-based practices' to cancer survivors and their families. In a recent national study of oncology social workers, findings revealed that these social workers faced numerous challenges in translating research into practice [333].

"I'm overloaded with my patients. I don't have time to read journal articles or search for information on the web. I would love to have the time to do this, but not in my world!"

The Association of Oncology Social Work (AOSW) (www.aosw.org) is one of the best places where oncology social workers can turn for information, professional development, and professional support. AOSW was created in 1984 by social workers interested in oncology and by existing national cancer organizations. They currently have over 1000 members who embrace the AOSW Mission "to advance excellence in the psychosocial care of persons with cancer, their families, and caregivers through networking, education, advocacy, research, and resource development." The membership comes from a variety of oncology settings: hospitals, outpatient clinics, home care and hospice agencies, community wellness programs, patient advocacy organizations, and other settings [25]. Oncology social workers can also find useful information on the websites of other oncology professional, such as the Oncology Nursing Society (www.ons.org) and the American Psychosocial Oncology Society (www.apos-society.org).

It is impossible for individual professionals to synthesize all the relevant literature in their field. Therefore, various organizations are dedicated to reviewing the large amounts of health care literature and providing professionals with systematic reviews of the literature. For example, a useful source of information for oncology social workers is the Cochrane Collaboration (http://www.cochrane.org/). The Cochrane Collaboration is an international not-for-profit and independent organization, dedicated to providing up-to-date, accurate information about the effects of health care readily available worldwide. It produces and disseminates systematic reviews of health care interventions and promotes the search for evidence in the form of clinical trials and other studies of interventions [334].

Attending professional conferences and continuing education programs are other strategies for oncology social workers to stay informed and up-to-date with the latest information. AOSW hosts an annual conference for oncology social workers, which is an excellent source of information and networking. In addition, the AOSW website provides links to other state, national, and international educational opportunities for oncology social workers as well as online continuing educational programs [1]. It is recommended that all oncology social workers join AOSW and become an active voice in this professional body.

Chapter 14

CHALLENGES AND FUTURE DIRECTIONS FOR ONCOLOGY SOCIAL WORK

"Social workers can play an important role, but not if patients don't know they're available. I was never told that a social worker was available to help me, and I was a single mother with two small children, no job, and no insurance when I was diagnosed with cancer."

The oncology social worker is an important part of the treatment team and a valuable resource to women with cancer, especially underserved women. However, the social work profession has some serious issues that need to be addressed in order to maintain their sustainability in the oncology world.

RESEARCH AGENDA

Evidence-based practice has become the gold standard in health care; yet, social workers have been slow to embrace this concept in their own professional domain. Evidence based practice and accountability are essential for professionals to survive in the health care setting.

An essential component to securing the future of oncology social work is the ability to demonstrate one's self worth and cost-effectiveness within the health care system. One obvious mechanism for accomplishing this goal is intervention based research, which clearly demonstrates the effectiveness of social workers on patient outcomes (e.g., an improvement in patients' psychological functioning, physical functioning, and quality of life) and/or cost-savings of oncology social workers.

Although some oncology social workers are engaged in research, the type of research being undertaken by and on social workers is often not intervention or outcome based research. In a study of research undertaken by medical social workers over a 10-year period, only five out of 44 studies were defined as "intervention" or "outcome" studies [335]. The majority of studies were either qualitative studies or quantitative studies that simply described what medical social workers are currently doing or how other professionals viewed social workers.

In order for oncology social workers to demonstrate their effectiveness both in terms of patient outcomes and cost-effectiveness, they must begin to engage in intervention or outcome based research. This type of research is the ideal mechanism through which oncology social workers can negotiate their position and value within the hospital setting. Examples of key research questions that need to be addressed are as follows:

- Are the interventions provided by oncology social workers effective in decreasing the psychological and/or physical problems experienced by survivors and their family members?
- Are the interventions provided by oncology social workers cost-effective to the health care system?
- Is one type of intervention more effective than another type of intervention? Under what conditions? With what type of patient?
- What are the direct and indirect benefits to having an oncology social worker as part of the treatment team?

Given the fact that oncology social workers already have full caseloads and are often over worked and stressed, the question becomes how can they be expected to undertake this level of research in addition to their already heavy caseloads? It is unrealistic to expect oncology social workers to have the time or training to design, implement, and analyze high quality intervention research.

"My supervisor in the social work department wants us to do research, but I don't have time and I don't really know where to begin. It's been years since I took a research class."

Therefore, we must be innovative in creating opportunities within the oncology setting for social workers to participate in this type of research.

One possible strategy is for social work departments to form partnerships with social work faculty and doctoral students who are interested in undertaking this type of research. This type of collaboration would be beneficial to both social workers in the academic setting and the oncology setting.

It is the primary responsibility of social work researchers to make these connections and develop appropriate studies for the oncology setting. Another possible strategy is for oncology social workers to become involved in current research and clinical trials being undertaken in the oncology setting by other health care professionals and researchers. Oncology social workers need to liaise and collaborate with these researchers regarding the possibility of assessing the effectiveness of social workers as part of their ongoing research. A final strategy is for the Association of Oncology Social Workers to take on this task as one of their priorities and provide funding or seek funding to implement this type of research on a large scale.

Many oncology social workers already collect valuable data on their patients, but without large numbers this information is not very useful. A national oncology social work database with systematic outcome data being collected on a large number of social work clients would be a great asset for the sustainability of the profession. Funding for this type of large-scale research study is more likely to be awarded as opposed to individual social work researcher grants. Regardless of the strategy, the important thing, given the current financial state of health care in this country, is that oncology social workers begin engaging in intervention or outcome based research.

CHALLENGES FROM OTHER PROFESSIONS

Currently, there is a shift toward the rationing of health care, and containing health care costs is a major issue for state and federal governments. Current economic rationing can have negative consequences for oncology social workers. Social workers seem to fit into the category of employees who are valued the least because they generate no revenue, their efficiency is not readily demonstrated, their cost-saving value is unmeasured, and their role is misunderstood or challenged [336]. Oncology social workers are being confronted with organizational restructuring, often resulting in the loss of social work positions in favor of "care coordinators" or "patient navigators". This has been attributed to various factors, including social workers' inability to articulate their value-added contributions, the hierarchy within the medical system, and role blurring with other medical professionals.

One of the reasons for this fight over "domain" is the lack of knowledge of what social workers do as part of the treatment team. Several studies have found role blurring and role conflict between nurses and social workers as well as the lack of knowledge among other professional about the role of social workers in the health care setting [337,338].

> "I agree with the need for a patient navigator, but if I'm going to hire someone in that position it is going to be a nurse. A nurse can do everything a social worker can, and she can provide medical care too."

Nurses currently overlap with oncology social workers in several key areas, such as conducting psychosocial assessments and providing supportive care.

> "It was the nurse who helped me arrange transportation and gave me resources for counseling. I only saw the social worker once in the hospital, but she didn't really help me."

Patient navigators are a very real threat to oncology social work positions. In a review of 11 patient navigation programs, Dohan and Schrag found that seven programs used lay workers while the other four used professionals, either nurses or social workers [30]. When describing the roles of patient navigators, these roles are consistent with the roles of the oncology social worker. The early patient navigator programs trained lay persons to be the patient navigator [26], and this model is still currently the dominant model, with patient navigator training programs developing across the country. If oncology social workers do not claim patient navigation as a social work domain, oncology social workers are at risk of losing a significant part of their role, which will ultimately result in a loss of funded positions for social workers. The social work profession must actively advocate for oncology social workers to fill the positions of patient navigators.

MEETING THE NEEDS OF MINORITY AND UNDERSERVED WOMEN

Unfortunately, many minority and underserved women are not getting the help they need from oncology social workers.

"I didn't see a social worker … this might be because I'm illegal in this country so I didn't get all the services."

There are several reasons for this including: lack of oncology social workers to serve vulnerable populations, lack of referrals from the medical team, resistance from survivors to access available social work services, lack of knowledge of how social workers can help, and language barriers.

"I never had a social worker help me, and I couldn't speak the language, but my church helped me."

Long-term survivorship brings new challenges for oncology social workers in the care of cancer survivors. A recent Institute of Medicine report, *Cancer Care for the Whole Patient: Meeting Psychosocial Needs*, emphasizes the importance of quality services along the full spectrum of the cancer care continuum [10]. In large part, oncology social workers have focused more on prevention, early detection strategies and the time period between diagnosis and treatment rather than how needs change across the continuum of care. Oncology social workers are generally based in settings that do not allow them to follow the patient from time of diagnosis into long-term survivorship.

"I saw a social worker in the hospital when I had my surgery, but I didn't see her again once I left the hospital. I didn't need her in the hospital, but I needed lots of help later on."

Thus, it is challenging for oncology social workers to provide continuity of care across the continuum of care.

One of the challenges for the social work profession is to develop new models of care to meet the changing needs of women with cancer over time.

"I want the social worker to come into my world and really see and understand my world. She needs to see me in my home to really understand me."

As demonstrated in the literature, the practical and emotional distress from the cancer experience does not end when the treatment ends. To the contrary, this is often the beginning of the long-term practical and emotional distress of cancer survivorship. Unfortunately, this is when survivors are least likely to be in contact with oncology social workers or other professionals to receive a referral to social work services.

"I don't want to go into some office and talk about my problems. I don't want another 'office' visit."

In order to truly meet the needs of women with cancer and their families, oncology social workers must provide their services throughout the entire cancer journey from time of diagnosis throughout the ups and downs of long-term survivorship and end-of-life.

"If you really want to help me, you need to know my story from beginning to end and be there with me along the way. It is hard to just meet someone for one or two times and expect them to understand how to help me."

It is the ethical responsibility of social workers to develop and test new models of care that meet the needs of underserved women with cancer and their families. If social workers are going to make real change in the delivery of services to this population, we need to have an active voice across all levels where decisions on service delivery are being made. This requires action from the front line oncology social workers providing care in hospitals, treatment centers, and community centers to social workers at the policy level bringing about change in the delivery of health care to cancer survivors and their families. Change in our health care system is inevitable. The challenge is to ensure that this change will meet the needs of the underserved. As said so eloquently by Margret Mead, "Never doubt that a small group of thoughtful, committed citizens can change the world; indeed, it's the only thing that ever has!"

APPENDIX A: SAMPLE RESOURCES FOR WOMEN WITH CANCER

Living Beyond Breast Cancer (LBBC)
610-645-4567
www.lbbc.org

Y-ME National Breast Cancer Organization
800-462-9273
www.y-me.org

National Coalition for Cancer Survivorship
877-6227937
www.canceradvocacy.org

Susan G. Komen Breast Cancer Foundation
800-462-9273
www.komen.org

SHARE: Self-Help for Women with Breast and Ovarian Cancer
866-891-2392
www.sharecancersupport.org

Sister's Network
713-781-0255
www.sistersnetworkinc.org

Young Survival Coalition
877-972-1011
www.youngsurvival.org

4th Angel Patient Mentor Program
216-445-8734
www.scottcares.com

FORCE: Facing Our Risk of Cancer Empowerment

866-288-7475
www.facingourrisk.org

CancerCare
800-813-4673
www.cancercare.org

The Wellness Community
888-793-9355
www.thewellnesscommunity.org

Gilda's Club
888-445-3248
www.gildasclub.org

Lance Armstrong Foundation
800-227-2345
www.livestrong.org

National Breast Cancer Coalition
800-622-2838
www.natlbcc.org

National Black Leadership Initiative on Cancer (NBLIC)
800-724-1185
www.nblic.org

Intercultural Cancer Council
713-798-4617
www.iccnetwork.org

American Cancer Society
800-277-2345
www.cancer.org

National Cancer Institute Cancer Information Services
800-4CANCER
www.cancer.gov

National Alliance for Hispanic Health
202-387-5000
www.hispanichealth.org

Mary-Helen Mautner Project for Lesbians with Cancer
202-332-5536
www.mautnerproject.org

APPENDIX B: SAMPLE RESOURCES FOR PARTNERS

Support and Information:

The American Association for Sex Educators, Counselors and Therapists
(www.AASECT.org)

Y-ME National Breast Cancer Organization
1-800-221-2141

Y-ME Men's Match Program
800-221-2141

Cancer Information Service of the National Cancer Institute
800-4-CANCER (1-800-422-6237)
http://cis.nci.nih.gov

National Coalition for Cancer Survivorship (NCCS)
301-650-8868
www.canceradvocacy.org

National Lymphedema Network
800-541-3259
www.lymphnet.org

Support Groups for Partners:

BreastCancer.org
www.breastcancer.org

The Mautner Project for Lesbians with Cancer
202-332-5536
www.mautnerproject.org

OncoChat
www.oncochat.org

Association of Cancer Online Resources
www.acor.org

Men Against Breast Cancer
(866) 547-MABC (866-547-6222)
www.menagainstbreastcancer.org

Well Spouse Foundation
1-800-838-0879
www.wellspouse.org

Sample Readings for Partners:

Breast Cancer Husband: How to Help Your Wife (and Yourself) Through Diagnosis, Treatment and Beyond
Mark Silver

Dr. Susan Love's Breast Book, 3rd Edition
Susan M. Love, M.D., with Karen Lindsey

Man to Man
Andy Murcia and Bob Stewart

Prayer, Laughter and Broccoli: Being There When Your Wife has Breast Cancer
Peter Flierl

Sexuality and Cancer: For the Woman Who Has Cancer and Her Partner
American Cancer Society

Taking Time: Support for People with Cancer and the People Who Care about Them
National Cancer Institute

When Life Becomes Precious: A Guide for Loved Ones and Friends of Cancer Patients
Elise Needell Babcock

APPENDIX C: SAMPLE RESOURCES FOR CHILDREN

Kids Konnected
800-899-2866
http://www.kidskonnected.org

The Children's Treehouse Foundation
303-322-1202
http://www.childrenstreehousefdn.org

CancerCare
800-813-4673
www.cancercare.org

The Wellness Community
888-793-9355
www.thewellnesscommunity.org

Gilda's Club
888-445-3248
www.gildasclub.org

American Cancer Society
1-800 ACS 2345
www.cancer.org

Books for kids:

- *After Diagnosis: A Guide for Patients and Families (also available in Spanish)*
- *It Helps To Have Friends When Mom or Dad Has Cancer*
- *When Your Brother or Sister Has Cancer*
- *Because Someone I Love Has Cancer: Kids' Activity Book.*
- *Cancer in the Family: Helping Children Cope with a Parent's Illness* by Sue P. Heiny, Joan F. Hermann, Katherine V. Bruss and Joy L. Fincannon.
- *Our Mom Has Cancer* by Adrienne Ackerman and Abigail Ackerman
- *Talking With My Treehouse Friends About Cancer* by Peter Van Dernoot

- *Lost and Found: A Kid's Book for Living Through Loss* by Marc Gellman and Debbie Tilley
- *In Mommy's Garden* by Neyal J. Ammary
- *My Mommy Has Cancer* by Carolyn S. Parkinson
- *Sammy's Mommy Has Cancer* by Sherry Kohlenberg
- *The Year My Mother Was Bald* by Ann Speltz and Kate Sternberg
- *When Your Parent has Cancer: A Guide for Teens* by the National Cancer Institute
- *Vanishing Cookies: Doing Ok When a Parent Has Cancer* by Michelle B. Goodman
- *Love Sick* by Kids Konnected

Books for adults:

- *Can I Still Kiss You? Answering Your Children's Questions About Cancer* by Neil Russell
- *Helping Your Children Cope With Your Cancer: A Guide for Parents (2nd Edition)* by Peter Van Dernoot
- *How to Help Children Through a Parent's Serious Illness* by Kathleen McCue and Ron Bonn
- *Life and Loss: A Guide to Help Grieving Children* by Linda Goldman
- *When a Parent Has Cancer: A Guide to Caring for Your Children* by Wendy S. Harpham
- *When Someone in Your Family Has Cancer* by the National Cancer Institute

ACKNOWLEDGMENTS

As with any major undertaking, it would not have been possible without a little help from my friends and family. I would first like to thank Dr. Kathleen Darby and Natalie Worley for their assistance in helping with the contents of this book. Their expertise was a valuable contribution to this book as well as their moral support. I would also like to thank my friend, Kelly Sweat, for her editorial critiques of this book, and Christy Collier and Catherine Wright for their assistance in various aspects of this project.

My children, Zak and Ali, deserve a special thank-you for their support and for sacrificing "mommy time" so that I could write this book. I would also like to thank my husband, Steve, and my mom who gave me time that I so desperately needed to get this project completed. As always, it was a family effort!

REFERENCES

[1] AOSW. About us <http://www.aosw.org/html/about.php>. Accessed 2008 April 30, 2008.

[2] Hoffman B, Stovall E. Survivorship perspectives and advocacy. *J. Clin. Oncol..* 2006 Nov 10;24(32):5154-9.

[3] Hewitt M, Greenfield S, Stovall E. From cancer patient to cancer survivor: Lost in transition. Washington, D.C.: Institute of Medicine and National Research Council, 2006.

[4] Ganz PA. Advocating for the woman with breast cancer. CA: *a cancer journal for clinicians.* 1995 Mar-Apr;45(2):114-26.

[5] Walsh-Burke K, Marcusen C. Self-advocacy training for cancer survivors. The Cancer Survival Toolbox. *Cancer practice.* 1999 Nov-Dec;7(6):297-301.

[6] American Academy of Nurse Practitioners. Frequently asked questions <http://npfinder.com/faq.pdf>. Accessed May 12, 2008, 2008.

[7] Ferrell BR, Grant M, Funk B, Otis-Green S, Garcia N. Quality of life in breast cancer. Part II: Psychological and spiritual well-being. *Cancer nursing.* 1998 Feb;21(1):1-9.

[8] Ferrell B, Grant M, Funk B, Otis-Green S, Garcia N. Quality of life in breast cancer. Part I: Physical and social well-being. *Cancer nursing.* 1997 Dec;20(6):398-408.

[9] Ferrell BR, Grant M, Funk B, Garcia N, Otis-Green S, Schaffner ML. Quality of life in breast cancer. *Cancer practice.* 1996 Nov-Dec;4(6):331-40.

[10] Institute of Medicine (IOM). Cancer care for the whole patient: Meeting psychosocial needs. Washington, D.C., 2007.

[11] Sharpe M, Strong V, Allen K, al. E. Major depression in outpatients attending a regional cancer centre: Screening and unmet treatment needs. *Br. J. Cancer.* 2004;90:314-20.

[12] American Psychosocial Oncology Society. APOS standards of care for the management of distress in patients with cancer. Charlottesville, VA: *American Psychosocial Oncology Society,* 2000.

[13] Fallowfield L, Ratcliffe D, Jenkins V, al. E. Psychiatric morbidity and its recognition by doctors in patients with cancer. *Br. J. Cancer.* 2001;84:1011-5.

[14] Mager WM, Andrykowski MA. Communication in the cancer 'bad news' consultation: patient perceptions and psychological adjustment. *Psycho-oncology.* 2002 Jan-Feb;11(1):35-46.

[15] Sollner W, DeVries A, Steixner E, al. E. How successful are oncologists in identifying patient distress, perceived social support, and need for psychosocial counseling? *Br. J. Cancer.* 2001;84:179-85.

[16] Rappaport J. Studies in empowerment: Introduction to the issue. *Prevention in Human Services.* 1984;3(2-3):1-7.

[17] Clark EJ, Stovall EL. Advocacy: the cornerstone of cancer survivorship. *Cancer practice.* 1996 Sep-Oct;4(5):239-44.

[18] Gray RE, Doan B, Church K. Empowerment issues in cancer. *Health Values.* 1991;15(4):22-8.

[19] Henderson P, Thomas DN. Skills in neighborhood work. 2nd ed. New York: Routledge; 1987.

[20] Clark E, Stovall E. Survivors as advocates. In: Hoffman B (ed). *A Cancer Survivor's Almanac.* New York: John Wiley, 2004:302-8.

[21] Stecher V, DeVillis B, Becker M, Rosenstock I. The role of self-efficacy in achieving health behavior change. *Health Education Quarterly.* 1986;13(1):73-92.

[22] McLeroy KR, Norton BL, Kegler MC, Burdine JN, Sumaya CV. Community-based interventions. *American journal of public health.* 2003 Apr;93(4):529-33.

[23] Itzhaky H, York AS. Empowerment and community participation: does gender make a difference? *Social Work Research.* 2000;24(4):225-34.

[24] Schriver JM. Human Behavior and the Social Environment. 4th ed. Boston: Pearson; 2004.

[25] Association of Oncology Social Work (AOSW). About us <http://www.aosw.org/html/about.php>. Accessed 2008 April 30, 2008.

[26] Freeman HP, Muth BJ, Kerner JF. Expanding access to cancer screening and clinical follow-up among the medically underserved. *Cancer practice.* 1995 Jan-Feb;3(1):19-30.

[27] LAF, CDC. A National Action Plan for Cancer Survivorship: *African American Priorities.* Washington, 2006. 15 p.

[28] Trans-HHS Cancer Health Disparities Progress Review Group. Making cancer health disparities history. Washington, D.C., 2004.

[29] Darnell JS. Patient navigation: a call to action. *Social work.* 2007 Jan;52(1):81-4.

[30] Dohan D, Schrag D. Using navigators to improve care of underserved patients: current practices and approaches. *Cancer.* 2005 Aug 15;104(4):848-55.

[31] Frelix GD, Rosenblatt R, Solomon M, Vikram B. Breast cancer screening in underserved women in the Bronx. *Journal of the National Medical Association.* 1999 Apr;91(4):195-200.

[32] Ell K, Vourlekis B, Muderspach L, et al. Abnormal cervical screen follow-up among low-income Latinas: Project SAFe. *Journal of women's health and gender-based medicine.* 2002 Sep;11(7):639-51.

[33] Weinrich SP, Boyd MD, Weinrich M, Greene F, Reynolds WA, Jr., Metlin C. Increasing prostate cancer screening in African American men with peer-educator and client-navigator interventions. *J. Cancer Educ.* 1998 Winter;13(4):213-9.

[34] Gardner C, Arya N, McAllister ML. Can a health unit take action on the determinants of health? *Can J. Public Health.* 2005 Sep-Oct;96(5):374-9.

[35] Rahm AK, Sukhanova A, Ellis J, Mouchawar J. Increasing utilization of cancer genetic counseling services using a patient navigator model. *J. Genet. Couns.* 2007 Apr;16(2):171-7.

[36] Weiss ME. Case management as a tool for clinical integration. *Adv. Pract. Nurs. Q.* 1998;4(1):9-15.

[37] Holloway F, Carson J. Review Article Case Management: an Update. *International Journal of Social Psychiatry.* 2001;47(3):21.

[38] Case Management Society of America (CMSA). Standards of Practice for Case Management, 2002.

[39] CDC. Cancer- Fast facts about breast cancer <http://www.cdc.gov/cancer/breast/>. Accessed 2008 March 6, 2008.

[40] American Cancer Society. Breast Cancer Facts and Figures 2007-2008. Atlanta, GA: *American Cancer Society*, 2007.

[41] Anastasia PJ, Bristow RE, Montz FJ. A guide to survivorship for women with ovarian cancer. Baltimore, MD: John Hopkins University Press; 2005.

[42] American Cancer Society. Home <http://www.cancer.org/docroot/home/index.asp>. Accessed 2008 March 31, 2008.

[43] American Cancer Society. Overview: Cervical Cancer <http://www.cancer.org/docroot/ CRI/CRI_2_1x.asp?rnav=criovanddt=8>. Accessed 2008 July 1. American Cancer Society, 2008.

[44] National Cancer Institute. Cervical Cancer <http://www.cancer.gov/cancertopics/ types/cervical>. Accessed 2008 July 9. National Cancer Institute, Washington, DC, 2008.

[45] Reproductive Health Outlook. Preventing cervical cancer: Unprecedented opportunities for improving women's health <http://www.rho.org/files/PATH_outlook23_1 _web.pdf>. Accessed 2008 May 29, 2007.

[46] American Cancer Society. Vaginal Cancer <http://www.cancer.org/docroot/CRI/ content/CRI_2_4_1X_What_is_vaginal_cancer_55.asp?sitearea=>. Accessed 2008 July 9. American Cancer Society, Washington, DC, 2008.

[47] American Cancer Society. Overview: Endometrial Cancer <http://www.cancer.org/ docroot/CRI/CRI_2_1x.asp?rnav=criovanddt=11>. Accessed 2008 July 1. American Cancer Society, 2008.

[48] National Cancer Institute. Endometrial Cancer <http://www.cancer.gov/ cancertopics/types/endometrial>. Accessed 2008 July 9. National Cancer Institute, Washington, DC, 2008.

[49] Ricks D. Breast cancer basics and beyond. Alameda, CA: Hunter House, Inc.; 2005.

[50] National Cancer Institute. Seer stat fact sheets- Cancer of the ovary <http://seer.cancer.gov/statfacts/html/ovary_print.html>. Accessed 2008 March 6, 2008.

[51] Conner K, Langford L. Ovarian cancer: Your guide to taking control. Sebastopol, CA: *O'Reilly and Associates*, Inc.; 2003.

[52] DeNavas-Walt C, Bernadette DP, Smith J. US Census Bureau Current Population Reports, P60-233 on Income, Poverty, and Health Insurance Coverage in the United States: 2006. Washington, DC: *US Census Bureau*, 2007.

[53] Jacobson JS, Grann VR, Hershman D, Troxel AB, Li H, Neugut AI. Breast biopsy and race/ethnicity among women without breast cancer. *Cancer detection and prevention.* 2006;30(2):129-33.

[54] Voti L, Richardson LC, Reis I, Fleming LE, Mackinnon J, Coebergh JW. The effect of race/ethnicity and insurance in the administration of standard therapy for local breast cancer in Florida. *Breast Cancer Res. Treat.* 2006 Jan;95(1):89-95.

[55] Judd S (ed). Breast cancer sourcebook. 2nd ed. Detroit, MI: *Omnigraphics*; 2004.

[56] Bach PB, Schrag D, Brawley OW, Galaznik A, Yakren S, Begg CB. Survival of blacks and whites after a cancer diagnosis. *JAMA*. 2002 April 24;287(16):2106-13.

[57] Freeman HP. Poverty, culture, and social injustice: Determinants of cancer disparities. CA: *a cancer journal for clinicians*. 2004 March 1, 2004;54(2):72-7.

[58] Tammemagi CM, Nerenz D, Neslund-Dudas C, Feldkamp C, Nathanson D. Comorbidity and survival disparities among black and white patients with breast cancer. *JAMA*. 2005 October 12;294(14):1765-72.

[59] Shavers VL, Brown ML. Racial and ethnic disparities in the receipt of cancer treatment. *Journal of the National Cancer Institute*. 2002 Mar 6;94(5):334-57.

[60] Newman LA, Griffith KA, Jatoi I, Simon MS, Crowe JP, Colditz GA. Meta-analysis of survival in african american and white american patients with breast cancer: Ethnicity compared with socioeconomic status. *J. Clin. Oncol.*. 2006 March 20;24(9):1342-9.

[61] Bickell NA, Chassin MR. Determining the quality of breast cancer care: do tumor registries measure up? *Ann. Intern. Med.* 2000 May 2;132(9):705-10.

[62] Blackman DJ, Masi CM. Racial and ethnic disparities in breast cancer mortality: Are we doing enough to address the root causes? *J. Clin. Oncol.*. 2006 May 10, 2006;24(14):2170-8.

[63] American Cancer Society. A breast cancer journey: Your personal guidebook. 2nd ed. Atlanta, GA: *American Cancer Society*; 2005.

[64] Saltzman BS, Doherty JA, Hill DA, et al. Diabetes and endometrial cancer: An evaluation of the modifying effects of other known risk factors. *American journal of epidemiology*. 2007;167(5):607-14.

[65] Phillips C. Alcohol and Breast Cancer Risk: New Findings NCI Cancer Bulletin. 2008;5(9):1.

[66] American Cancer Society. Cancer Facts and Figures 2006 <www.cancer.org/downloads/stt/CAFFO6EsCsSt.pdf>. Accessed 2008 July 15. American Cancer Society, 2006.

[67] Au WW. Life style, environmental and genetic susceptibility to cervical cancer. *Toxicology*. 2004 May 20;198(1-3):117-20.

[68] Mayo Clinic. Genetic testing for colon cancer: Should you consider it? <http://www.mayoclinic.com/health/colon-cancer/HQ00448>. Accessed 2008 May, 29, 2007.

[69] Sonoda Y, Barakat RR. Screening and the prevention of gynecologic cancer: endometrial cancer. Best Pract Res Clin Obstet Gynaecol. 2006 Apr;20(2):363-77.

[70] American College of Obstetricians and Gynecologists. Human Papilloma Virus Infection <http://www.acog.org/publications/patient_education/bp073.cfm>. Accessed 2008 June 2, 2006.

[71] Mechcatie E. HPV vaccine wins strong support (human papilloma virus). *Internal Medicine News*. 2006;39(12):1-2.

[72] Mayo Clinic. Cervical Cancer <http://www.mayoclinic.com/health/cervical-cancer/DS00167/DSECTION=risk-factors>. Accessed 2008 June, 2, 2007.

[73] Walling AD. Endometrial cancer risk after tamoxifen therapy. *American Family Physician.* 2001;63(6):1204-6.

[74] Northouse P, Northouse N. Communication and cancer: Issues confronting patients, health professionals, and family members. *Journal of psychosocial oncology.* 1987;5(3):17-46.

[75] Northouse L. The family impact of cancer in women. Third National Conference on *Cancer Nursing Research*, Newport Beach, CA, Jan. 1994:27–9.

[76] Avis NE, Crawford S, Manuel J. Quality of life among younger women with breast cancer. *J. Clin. Oncol..* 2005 May 20;23(15):3322-30.

[77] Manuel JC, Burwell SR, Crawford SL, et al. Younger women's perceptions of coping with breast cancer. *Cancer nursing.* 2007 Mar-Apr;30(2):85-94.

[78] Coyne E, Borbasi S. Holding it all together: breast cancer and its impact on life for younger women. *Contemp Nurse.* 2006 Dec-2007 Jan;23(2):157-69.

[79] Avis NE, Crawford S, Manuel J. Psychosocial problems among younger women with breast cancer. *Psycho-oncology.* 2004 May;13(5):295-308.

[80] Allen S, Shah, A., Nezu, A., Nezu, C., Ciambrone, D., Hogan, J., and Mor, V. . A problem-solving approach to stress reduction among younger women with breast carcinoma: A randomized controlled trial. *Cancer.* 2002;94(12):11.

[81] Wenzel LB, Fairclough DL, Brady MJ, et al. Age-related differences in the quality of life of breast carcinoma patients after treatment. Cancer. 1999 Nov 1;86(9):1768-74.

[82] Dunn J, Steginga SK. Young women's experience of breast cancer: defining young and identifying concerns. *Psycho-oncology.* 2000 Mar-Apr;9(2):137-46.

[83] Mastro L, Catzeddu T, Venturini M. Infertility and pregnancy after breast cancer: Current knowledge and future perspectives. *Cancer treatment reviews.* 2006;32:417-22.

[84] Blakely LJ, Buzdar AU, Lozada JA, et al. Effects of pregnancy after treatment for breast carcinoma on survival and risk of recurrence. *Cancer.* 2004 Feb 1;100(3):465-9.

[85] Velentgas P, Daling JR, Malone KE, et al. Pregnancy after breast carcinoma: outcomes and influence on mortality. *Cancer.* 1999 Jun 1;85(11):2424-32.

[86] Kroman N, Jensen MB, Wohlfahrt J, Mouridsen HT, Andersen PK, Melbye M. Factors influencing the effect of age on prognosis in breast cancer: population based study. *British Medical Journal.* 2000 Feb 19;320(7233):474-8.

[87] Susan G. Komen Cancer Foundation. Factsheet: Young women and breast cancer <http://www.komen.org/stellent/groups/harvard_group/@dallas/documents/-komen _site_documents/spbcyoung.pdf.>. Accessed June 4, 2007, 2006.

[88] Sampson D. Race Influences Uterine Cancer Survival. Atlanta, 2006.

[89] ACS. Breast Cancer Facts and Figures for African Americans. Atlanta: ACS, 2003.

[90] Jacobellis J, Cutter G. Mammography screening and differences in stage of disease by race/ethnicity. *American journal of public health.* 2002 Jul;92(7):1144-50.

[91] O'Malley CD, Le GM, Glaser SL, Shema SJ, West DW. Socioeconomic status and breast carcinoma survival in four racial/ethnic groups: a population-based study. *Cancer.* 2003 Mar 1;97(5):1303-11.

[92] Halpern MT, Schrag NM, Ward EM, Chen AY, Bian J. Insurance status and stage of cancer at diagnosis among women with breast cancer. *Cancer.* 2007 110(2):403-11.

[93] Lannin DR, Mathews HF, Mitchell J, Swanson MS, Swanson FH, Edwards MS. Influence of socioeconomic and cultural factors on racial differences in late-stage

presentation of breast cancer. *Journal of the American Medical Association.* 1998 Jun 10;279(22):1801-7.

[94] Lannin DR, Mathews HF, Mitchell J, Swanson MS. Impacting cultural attitudes in African-American women to decrease breast cancer mortality. *American journal of surgery.* 2002 Nov;184(5):418-23.

[95] Breen N, Kessler LG, Brown ML. Breast cancer control among the underserved--an overview. *Breast Cancer Res. Treat.* 1996;40(1):105-15.

[96] Aziz NM, Rowland JH. Cancer survivorship research among ethnic minority and medically underserved groups. *Oncology nursing forum.* 2002 Jun;29(5):789-801.

[97] Richardson LC. Treatment of breast cancer in medically underserved women: a review. *The breast journal.* 2004 Jan-Feb;10(1):2-5.

[98] Wolff M, Bates T, Beck B, Young S, Ahmed SM, Maurana C. Cancer prevention in underserved African American communities: barriers and effective strategies--a review of the literature. *Wisconsin Medical Journal.* 2003;102(5):36-40.

[99] Mandelblatt JS, Gold K, O'Malley MS, et al. Breast and cervix cancer screening among multiethnic women: Role of age, health and usual source of care. *Prev. Med.* 1999;28:418-25.

[100] Weinick RM, Zuvekas SH. Experience of primary care by racial and ethnic groups. *Med. Care.* 2000 Apr;38(4):447-8.

[101] Husaini BA, Sherkat DE, Bragg R, et al. Predictors of breast cancer screening in a panel study of African American women. *Women and health.* 2001;34(3):35-51.

[102] Davis C, Emerson JS, Husaini BA. Breast cancer screening among African American women: adherence to current recommendations. *Journal of health care for the poor and underserved.* 2005 May;16(2):308-14.

[103] Lantz PM, Reding D. Cancer: beliefs and attitudes of migrant Latinos. *Journal of the American Medical Association.* 1994 Jul 6;272(1):31-2.

[104] Lantz PM, Dupuis L, Reding D, Krauska M, Lappe K. Peer discussions of cancer among Hispanic migrant farm workers. *Public Health Rep.* 1994 Jul-Aug;109(4):512-20.

[105] Ramirez AG, McAlister A, Gallion KJ, Villarreal R. Targeting Hispanic populations: future research and prevention strategies. *Environ Health Perspect.* 1995 Nov;103 Suppl 8:287-90.

[106] Holm CJ, Frank DI, Curtin J. Health beliefs, health locus of control, and women's mammography behavior. *Cancer nursing.* 1999 Apr;22(2):149-56.

[107] Vernon SW, Vogel VG, Halabi S, Jackson GL, Lundy RO, Peters GN. Breast cancer screening behaviors and attitudes in three racial/ethnic groups. *Cancer.* 1992 Jan 1;69(1):165-74.

[108] Rojas M, Mandelblatt J, Cagney K, Kerner J, Freeman H. Barriers to follow-up of abnormal screening mammograms among low-income minority women. Cancer Control Center of Harlem. *Ethn Health.* 1996 Sep;1(3):221-8.

[109] Crump SR, Mayberry RM, Taylor BD, Barefield KP, Thomas PE. Factors related to noncompliance with screening mammogram appointments among low-income African-American women. *Journal of the National Medical Association.* 2000 May;92(5):237-46.

[110] Bowen D, Hickman KM, Powers D. Importance of psychological variables in understanding risk perceptions and breast cancer screening of African American women. *Women's health* (Hillsdale, NJ. 1997 Fall-Winter;3(3-4):227-42.

[111] Kang SH, Bloom JR, Romano PS. Cancer screening among African-American women: their use of tests and social support. *American journal of public health.* 1994 Jan;84(1):101-3.

[112] Brown G. Carin' and sharin' breast cancer education and support group. 24th Annual Conference of the Association of Oncology Social Work. Louisville, KY: *AOSW*, 2008.

[113] Ries LAG, Melbert D KM, Mariotto A, Miller BA, Feuer EJ, Clegg L, Horner MJ, Howlader N, Eisner MP, Reichman M, Edwards BK (eds). SEER Cancer Statistics Review, 1975-2004. Bethesda, MD: National Cancer Institute; 2000. Available from http://seer.cancer.gov/csr/1975_2004/, based on November 2006 SEER data submission, posted to the SEER web site, 2007.

[114] American Cancer Society. Cancer Facts and Figures for Hispanics/ Latinos <http://www.cancer.org/downloads/STT/CAFF2006HispPWSecured.pdf>. Accessed 2008 June 15. *American Cancer Society*, 2006.

[115] Li CI, Malone KE, Daling JR. Differences in breast cancer stage, treatment, and survival by race and ethnicity. . Arch Intern Med. 2003 163(1):49-56.

[116] Gilliland FD HW, Key CR. Trends in the survival of American Indian, Hispanic, and Non-Hispanic White cancer patients in New Mexico and Arizona, 1969-1994. *Cancer.* 1998;82(9):1769-83.

[117] Ramirez AG SL, McAlister A, Villarreal R, Trapido E, Talavera GA, Pérez-Stable E, Marti J. Cervical cancer screening in regional Hispanic populations. *Am. J. Health Behav.* 2000; 24(3):181-92.

[118] Ashing-Giwa K, Padilla, GV, Bohorquez, DE, Tejero, JS, Garcia, M. Understanding the breast cancer experience of Latina women. *Journal of psychosocial oncology.* 2006;24(3):19-52.

[119] Ramirez AG TG, Villarreal R, Suarez L, McAlister A, Trapido E, Pérez-Stable E, and Marti J. Breast cancer screening in regional Hispanic populations. *Health Educ. Res.* 2000;15(5):559-68.

[120] Ramirez AG MA, Gallion K, Villarreal R. Targeting Hispanic populations: future research and prevention strategies. *Environ. Health Perspect* 1995;103(8 Suppl):287-90.

[121] Ramirez AG SL, Laufman L, Barroso C, Chalela P. Hispanic women's breast and cervical cancer knowledge, attitudes and screening behaviors. *Am. J. Health Promot.* 2000;14(5):292-300.

[122] US Department of Health and Human Services. Racial and ethnic disparities in health. <http://raceandhealth.hhs.gov/3rdpgBlue/Cancer/3pgGoalsCancer.htm>. Accessed, 1998.

[123] US Census Bureau. The Hispanic population in the United States: 1999 <http://www.census.gov/prod/2000pubs/p20-527.pdf.>. Accessed, Washington, DC, 2000.

[124] American College of Physicians – American Society of Internal Medicine. No health insurance? It's enough to make you sick. Latino community at great risk. . College of Physicians – *American Society of Internal Medicine-American Society of Internal Medicine*; White Paper 2000.

[125] Schettino MR, Hernandez-Valero MA, Moguel R, Hajek RA, Jones LA. Assessing breast cancer knowledge, beliefs, and misconceptions among Latinas in Houston, Texas. *J. Cancer. Educ.* 2006 Spring;21(1 Suppl):S42-6.

[126] Morgan C, Park E, Cortes D. Beliefs, knowledge, and behavior about cancer among urban Hispanic women. *J. Natl. Cancer Inst. Monogr.* 1995;19(18):57-63.

[127] Hubbell FA, Valdez RB, Chavez LR, Mishra SI. Differing beliefs about breast cancer among Latinas and Anglo women. *West J. Med.* 1996 164(5):405-9.

[128] Howard AF, Balneaves LG, Bottorff JL. Ethnocultural women's experiences of breast cancer: a qualitative meta-study. *Cancer nursing.* 2007 Jul-Aug;30(4):E27-35.

[129] Cox C, Kelly D, Talman K, Coutts A. 'Human Cost' of breast cancer among non-English speaking BME women. *Cancer Nursing Practice.* 2007;6(6):31-5.

[130] Glanz K, Croyle RT, Chollette VY, Pinn VW. Cancer-related health disparities in women. *American journal of public health.* 2003 Feb;93(2):292-8.

[131] Dow Meneses K, Yarbro CH. Cultural perspectives of international breast health and breast cancer education. *J. Nurs. Scholarsh.* 2007;39(2):105-12.

[132] Azaiza F, Cohen M. Health beliefs and rates of breast cancer screening among Arab women. *Journal of women's health* (2002). 2006 Jun;15(5):520-30.

[133] Chou FY, Dodd M, Abrams D, Padilla G. Symptoms, self-care, and quality of life of Chinese American patients with cancer. *Oncology nursing forum.* 2007 Nov;34(6):1162-7.

[134] Intercultural Cancer Council. *Native Hawaiians and Pacific Islanders and Cancers.* Houston, TX, 2004.

[135] Miller BA, Chu KC, Hankey BF, Ries LA. Cancer incidence and mortality patterns among specific Asian and Pacific Islander populations in the U.S. *Cancer Causes Control.* 2008 Apr;19(3):227-56.

[136] Intercultural Cancer Council. *American Indians/Alaska Natives and Cancer.* Houston, TX, 2004.

[137] Intercultural Cancer Council. *Asian Americans and Cancer.* Houston, TX, 2004.

[138] Ashing-Giwa KT, Kagawa-Singer M, Padilla GV, et al. The impact of cervical cancer and dysplasia: a qualitative, multiethnic study. *Psycho-oncology.* 2004 Oct;13(10):709-28.

[139] Harle MT, Dela RF, Veloso G, Rock J, Faulkner J, Cohen MZ. The experiences of Filipino American patients with cancer. *Oncology nursing forum.* 2007 Nov; 34(6):1170-5.

[140] Bettencourt BA, Schlegel RJ, Talley AE, Molix LA. The breast cancer experience of rural women: a literature review. *Psycho-oncology.* 2007 Oct;16(10):875-87.

[141] Wingo PA, Tucker TC, Jamison PM, et al. *Cancer in Appalachia,* 2001-2003. Altanta, 2007.

[142] Ell K, Xie B, Wells A, Nedjat-Haiem F, Lee PJ, Vourlekis B. Economic stress among low-income women with cancer: Effects on quality of life. Atlanta, 2007.

[143] Tropman SE, Ricketts TC, Paskett E, Hatzell TA, Cooper MR, Aldrich T. Rural breast cancer treatment: evidence from the Reaching Communities for Cancer Care (REACH) project. *Breast Cancer Res. Treat.* 1999 Jul;56(1):59-66.

[144] Gray RE, James P, Manthorne J, Gould J, Fitch MI. A consultation with Canadian rural women with breast cancer. *Health Expect.* 2004 Mar;7(1):40-50.

[145] Howe HL, Katterhagen JG, Yates J, Lehnherr M. Urban-rural differences in the management of breast cancer. *Cancer Causes Control*. 1992 Nov;3(6):533-9.

[146] Hatzell TA, Ricketts TC, Tropman SE, Paskett ED, Cooper MR. Rural physicians' understanding of the state-of-the-art in breast, colon and rectum cancer treatment. *Cancer Causes Control*. 1999 Aug;10(4):261-7.

[147] Dunaway FW, Hueston WJ, Clevinger L. An exploratory study of the experiences of rural women with breast cancer. *J. Ky Med. Assoc.* 1995 Jun;93(6):241-5.

[148] Davis C, Girgis A, Williams P, Beeney L. Needs assessment of rural and remote women travelling to the city for breast cancer treatment. *Australian and New Zealand journal of public health*. 1998 Aug;22(5):525-7.

[149] Wilson SE, Andersen MR, Meischke H. Meeting the needs of rural breast cancer survivors: what still needs to be done? *Journal of women's health and gender-based medicine*. 2000 Jul-Aug;9(6):667-77.

[150] McGrath P, Patterson C, Yates P, Treloar S, Oldenburg B, Loos C. A study of postdiagnosis breast cancer concerns for women living in rural and remote Queensland. Part II: Support issues. *Aust. J. Rural Health*. 1999 Feb;7(1):43-52.

[151] McGrath P, Patterson C, Yates P, Treloar S, Oldenburg B, Loos C. A study of postdiagnosis breast cancer concerns for women living in rural and remote Queensland. Part I: Personal concerns. *Aust. J. Rural Health*. 1999 Feb;7(1):34-42.

[152] Rogers-Clark C. Living with breast cancer: the influence of rurality on women's suffering and resilience. a postmodern feminist inquiry. *Aust. J. Adv. Nurs*. 2002 Dec-2003 Feb;20(2):34-9.

[153] Demaree A. The interrelationships among social support satisfaction, functional impairment, prognosis, and depression in a rural sample of cancer patients undergoing radiation therapy. *Dissertation Abstracts International*. 2000;60:6358.

[154] National Cancer Institute. When Someone You Love Has Advanced Cancer. Bethesda, MD: *National Cancer Institute*, 2006 2006. Report No.: 06-5727.

[155] Johnson SM. Fears about breast cancer recurrence: Interviews with a diverse sample. Cancer practice. 2001;9(5):237-43.

[156] Shaffer A. Facing the future: Coping with fear of recurrence. <http://www.lbbc.org/content/newsletter-article/facing-the-future-coping-with-fear-of-recurrence.asp?section_tag=G>. Accessed. Living Beyond Breast Cancer, 2006.

[157] National Cancer Institute. When Cancer Returns. Washington, DC, 2005 August. Report No.: 05-2709.

[158] Ptacek JT, Ptacek JJ. Patients' perceptions of receiving bad news about cancer. *J. Clin. Oncol*. 2001 Nov 1;19(21):4160-4.

[159] Ptacek JT, Fries EA, Eberhardt TL, Ptacek JJ. Breaking bad news to patients: physicians' perceptions of the process. *Support Care Cancer*. 1999 May;7(3):113-20.

[160] Butow PN, Dowsett S, Hagerty R, Tattersall MH. Communicating prognosis to patients with metastatic disease: what do they really want to know? *Support Care Cancer*. 2002 Mar;10(2):161-8.

[161] Clayton JM, Butow PN, Tattersall MH. The needs of terminally ill cancer patients versus those of caregivers for information regarding prognosis and end-of-life issues. *Cancer*. 2005 May 1;103(9):1957-64.

[162] Hagerty RG, Butow PN, Ellis PM, Dimitry S, Tattersall MH. Communicating prognosis in cancer care: a systematic review of the literature. *Ann. Oncol.* 2005 Jul;16(7):1005-53.

[163] Lobb EA, Kenny DT, Butow PN, Tattersall MH. Women's preferences for discussion of prognosis in early breast cancer. *Health Expect.* 2001 Mar;4(1):48-57.

[164] Lobb EA, Butow PN, Meiser B, et al. Women's preferences and consultants' communication of risk in consultations about familial breast cancer: impact on patient outcomes. *J. Med. Genet.* 2003 May;40(5):e56.

[165] Gattellari M, Voigt KJ, Butow PN, Tattersall MH. When the treatment goal is not cure: are cancer patients equipped to make informed decisions? *J. Clin. Oncol.* 2002 Jan 15;20(2):503-13.

[166] Hagerty RG, Butow PN, Ellis PA, et al. Cancer patient preferences for communication of prognosis in the metastatic setting. *J. Clin. Oncol.* 2004 May 1;22(9):1721-30.

[167] Steinhauser KE, Christakis NA, Clipp EC, McNeilly M, McIntyre L, Tulsky JA. Factors considered important at the end of life by patients, family, physicians, and other care providers. *JAMA.* 2000 Nov 15;284(19):2476-82.

[168] Hagerty RG, Butow PN, Ellis PM, et al. Communicating with realism and hope: incurable cancer patients' views on the disclosure of prognosis. *J. Clin. Oncol.* 2005 Feb 20;23(6):1278-88.

[169] Christakis NA, Lamont EB. Extent and determinants of error in doctors' prognoses in terminally ill patients: prospective cohort study. *BMJ* (Clinical research ed. 2000 Feb 19;320(7233):469-72.

[170] Bradley EH, Hallemeier AG, Fried TR, et al. Documentation of discussions about prognosis with terminally ill patients. *Am. J. Med.* 2001 Aug 15;111(3):218-23.

[171] Pier TJ, Ahmed K. Difficult Conversations: Preparation for End-of-Life Decision Making. 24th Annual Conference of the Association of Oncology Social Work. Louisville, KY: AOSW, 2008.

[172] Otis-Green S. ACE Project - Advocating for Clinical Excellence: Transdisciplinary Palliative Care Education. 24th Annual Conference of the Association of Oncology Social Work. Louisville, KY: AOSW, 2008.

[173] Brandt AM, Gardner M. Antagonism and accommodation: interpreting the relationship between public health and medicine in the United States during the 20th century. *American journal of public health.* 2000 May;90(5):707-15.

[174] Allen AT. Reformers and radicals. *Journal of Urban History.* 2007;34(1):139-44.

[175] Treadwell K, Cram N. Managed Healthcare and federal health programs. *Journal of Clinical Engineering.* 2004;29(1):36-42.

[176] Kongstvedt PR. The Managed Care Health Care Handbook. 3rd ed. Gaitherburg, MD: *Aspen Publishers* Inc; 1996.

[177] Cohn J. The Untold Story of America's Health Care Crisis—and the People Who Pay the Price. New York: *HarperCollins Publishers*; 2007.

[178] Farlex. The Free Dictionary: Health Care <http://legal-dictionary.thefreedictionary.com/Health+benefits>. Accessed 2008 July 14. Farlex, Inc., 2008.

[179] Robinson JC. The end of managed care. *JAMA.* 2001 May 23-30;285(20):2622-8.

[180] Kaiser Family Foundation. Key Factors: Race, *Ethnicity and Medical Care.* Menlo Park, CA, 2007.

[181] Kaiser Family Foundation. Employee Health Benefits: 2007 *Annual Survey*. Menlo Park, CA, 2006 September.

[182] Agency for Healthcare and Research and Quality. Health care cost and financing: The financial burden of health care for people under age 65 increased between 1996 and 2003. Washington, DC, 2007. Report No.: 07-R022.

[183] Short PF, Banthin JS. New estimates of the underinsured younger than 65 years. *JAMA*. 1995 Oct 25;274(16):1302-6.

[184] Banthin JS, Bernard DM. Changes in financial burdens for health care: national estimates for the population younger than 65 years, 1996 to 2003. *JAMA*. 2006 Dec 13;296(22):2712-9.

[185] Kressin NR. Separate but not equal: the consequences of segregated health care. *Circulation*. 2005 Oct 25;112(17):2582-4.

[186] Smedley BD, Stith AY, Nelson AR (eds). Unequal Treatment: Confronting Racial and Ethnic Disparties in Health Care. Washington, DC: Institute of Medicine; 2003.

[187] Agency for Healthcare and Research and Quality. Key themes and highlights from the National Healthcare Disparities Report <http://www.ahrq.gov/qual/nhdr07/Key.htm>. Accessed 2008 July 1. U.S. *Department of Health and Human Services*, Washington, DC, 2007.

[188] Taylor AK, Larson S, Correa-de-Araujo R. Women's health care utilization and expenditures. *Womens Health Issues*. 2006 Mar-Apr;16(2):66-79.

[189] Ayanian JZ, Kohler BA, Abe T, Epstein AM. The relation between health insurance coverage and clinical outcomes among women with breast cancer. *The New England journal of medicine*. 1993 Jul 29;329(5):326-31.

[190] Richardson LC, Schulman J, Sever LE, Lee NC, Coate RJ. Early-stage breast cancer treatment among medically underserved women diagnosed in a national screening program, 1992-1995. *Breast Cancer Res. Treat*. 2001 Sep;69(2):133-42.

[191] Liu MJ, Hawk H, Gershman ST, et al. The effects of a National Breast and Cervical Cancer Early Detection Program on social disparities in breast cancer diagnosis and treatment in Massachusetts. *Cancer Causes Control*. 2005 Feb;16(1):27-33.

[192] Coburn N, Fulton J, Pearlman DN, Law C, DiPaolo B, Cady B. Treatment variation by insurance status for breast cancer patients. *The breast journal*. 2008 Mar-Apr;14(2):128-34.

[193] O'Hara B. Do medical out-of-pocket expenses thrust families into poverty? *Journal of health care for the poor and underserved*. 2004 Feb;15(1):63-75.

[194] Arozullah AM, Calhoun EA, Wolf M, et al. The financial burden of cancer: estimates from a study of insured women with breast cancer. *J. Support Oncol*. 2004 May-Jun;2(3):271-8.

[195] Intercultural Cancer Council. *Pain and Cancer*. Houston, TX, 2003.

[196] Intercultural Cancer Council. *Fatigue and Cancer*. Houston, TX, 2005.

[197] Stanton AL. Psychosocial concerns and interventions for cancer survivors. *J. Clin. Oncol*. 2006 Nov 10;24(32):5132-7.

[198] Michael YL, Kawaci I, Berkman LF, Holmes MD, Colditz GA. The persistent impact of breast carcinoma on functional health status: Prospective evidence from the nurses health study. *Cancer*. 2000;89(11):2176-86.

[199] Carver CS, Pozo C, Harris SD, et al. How coping mediates the effect of optimism on distress: a study of women with early stage breast cancer. *J. Pers. Soc. Psychol.* 1993 Aug;65(2):375-90.

[200] Hegel MT, Moore CP, Collins ED, et al. Distress, psychiatric syndromes, and impairment of function in women with newly diagnosed breast cancer. *Cancer.* 2006 Dec 15;107(12):2924-31.

[201] Mitchell AJ. Accuracy of distress thermometer and other ultra-short methods of detecting cancer-related mood disorders: Pooled results from 38 analyses. *J. Clin. Oncol.* 2007 October 10;25(29):1-12.

[202] Sanson-Fisher R, Girgis A, Boyes A, Bonevski B, Burton L, Cook P. The unmet supportive care needs of patients with cancer. Supportive Care Review Group. *Cancer.* 2000 Jan 1;88(1):226-37.

[203] Stanton AL, Snider PR. Coping with a breast cancer diagnosis: a prospective study. *Health Psychol.* 1993 Jan;12(1):16-23.

[204] Zabora J, BrintzenhofeSzoc K, Curbow B, Hooker C, Piantadosi S. The prevalence of psychological distress by cancer site. *Psycho-oncology.* 2001 Jan-Feb;10(1):19-28.

[205] Andrykowski MA, Carpenter JS, Studts JL, et al. Psychological impact of benign breast biopsy: a longitudinal, comparative study. *Health Psychol.* 2002 Sep;21(5):485-94.

[206] Coyne JC, Palmer SC, Shapiro PJ, Thompson R, DeMichele A. Distress, psychiatric morbidity, and prescriptions for psychotropic medication in a breast cancer waiting room sample. *General hospital psychiatry.* 2004 Mar-Apr;26(2):121-8.

[207] Ahles TA, Saykin AJ, Furstenberg CT, et al. Quality of life of long-term survivors of breast cancer and lymphoma treated with standard-dose chemotherapy or local therapy. *J. Clin. Oncol.* 2005 Jul 1;23(19):4399-405.

[208] Kornblith AB, Herndon JE, 2nd, Weiss RB, et al. Long-term adjustment of survivors of early-stage breast carcinoma, 20 years after adjuvant chemotherapy. *Cancer.* 2003 Aug 15;98(4):679-89.

[209] Spiegel D, Morrow GR, Classen C, et al. Group psychotherapy for recently diagnosed breast cancer patients: a multicenter feasibility study. *Psycho-oncology.* 1999 Nov-Dec;8(6):482-93.

[210] Heim E, Valach L, Schaffner L. Coping and psychosocial adaptation: longitudinal effects over time and stages in breast cancer. *Psychosom. Med.* 1997 Jul-Aug;59(4):408-18.

[211] Ganz PA, Hirji K, Sim MS, Schag CA, Fred C, Polinsky ML. Predicting psychosocial risk in patients with breast cancer. *Med. Care.* 1993 May;31(5):419-31.

[212] Blake-Mortimer J, Gore-Felton C, Kimerling R, Turner-Cobb JM, Spiegel D. Improving the quality and quantity of life among patients with cancer: a review of the effectiveness of group psychotherapy. *Eur. J. Cancer.* 1999 Oct;35(11):1581-6.

[213] Ganz PA, Kwan L, Stanton AL, et al. Quality of life at the end of primary treatment of breast cancer: First results from the moving beyond cancer randomized trial. *J. Natl. Cancer Inst.* 2004 March 3, 2004;96(5):376-87.

[214] Graves KD. Social cognitive theory and cancer patients' quality of life: a meta-analysis of psychosocial intervention components. *Health Psychol.* 2003 Mar;22(2):210-9.

[215] McCaul KD, Sandgren AK, King B, O'Donnell S, Branstetter A, Foreman G. Coping and adjustment to breast cancer. *Psycho-oncology.* 1999 May-Jun;8(3):230-6.

[216] Patrick-Miller LJ, Broccoli TL, Much JK, Levine E. Validation of the distress thermometer: A single item screen to detect clinically significant psychological distress in ambulatory oncology patients. *J. Clin. Oncol.* 2004;22(14, Suppl.):6024.

[217] Schnoll RA, Harlow LL, Stolbach LL, Brandt U. A structural model of the relationships among stage of disease, age, coping, and psychological adjustment in women with breast cancer. *Psycho-oncology.* 1998 Mar-Apr;7(2):69-77.

[218] Stanton AL, Danoff-Burg S, Cameron CL, et al. Emotionally expressive coping predicts psychological and physical adjustment to breast cancer. *J. Consult Clin. Psychol.* 2000 Oct;68(5):875-82.

[219] Rowland JH, Hewitt M, Ganz PA. Cancer survivorship: a new challenge in delivering quality cancer care. *J. Clin. Oncol.* 2006 Nov 10;24(32):5101-4.

[220] Rowland JH. Survivorship research: Past, present, and future. In: Chang AE, Ganz PA, Hayes DF, et al. (eds). Oncology: An Evidence Based Approach. New York, NY: Springer, 2006:1753.

[221] Hewitt M, Herdman R, Holland J (eds). Meeting the Psychosocial Needs of Women with Breast Cancer: National Cancer Policy Board Washington DC: The National Academic Press; 2004.

[222] O'Hair D, Villagran MM, Wittenberg E, et al. Cancer survivorship and agency model: implications for patient choice, decision making, and influence. *Health Commun.* 2003;15(2):193-202.

[223] Stovall E. Cancer advocacy. In: Chang AE, Ganz PA, Hayes DF, et al. (eds). Oncology: An Evidence based Approach. New York, NY: Springer, 2006:1955.

[224] Lerman C, Daly M, Walsh WP, et al. Communication between patients with breast cancer and health care providers. Determinants and implications. Cancer. 1993 Nov 1;72(9):2612-20.

[225] Foley G. Everybody's talking, not communicating. *Cancer practice.* 1995 Mar-Apr;3(2):71.

[226] Stanton AL, Reed GM. The breast cancer notebook: The healing power of reflection. Washington, D.C.: *American Psychological Association*; 2003.

[227] Burke S, Kissane DW. Psychosocial impact of breast cancer: A review of interventions by specialist providers. Australia, 1998.

[228] Arnold EM. The cessation of cancer treatment as a crisis. *Social work in health care.* 1999;29(2):21-38.

[229] Cappiello M, Cunningham RS, Knobf MT, Erdos D. Breast cancer survivors: information and support after treatment. *Clin. Nurs. Res.* 2007 Nov;16(4):278-93; discussion 94-301.

[230] Underwood SM. Research institute for nurse scientists responds to the challenge to expand and strengthen research focused on breast cancer in African American women. *Cancer.* 2007 Jan 15;109(2 Suppl):396-405.

[231] Mullan F. Seasons of survival: reflections of a physician with cancer. *The New England journal of medicine.* 1985 Jul 25;313(4):270-3.

[232] Pollack LA, Greer GE, Rowland JH, et al. Cancer survivorship: a new challenge in comprehensive cancer control. *Cancer Causes Control.* 2005 Oct;16 Suppl 1:51-9.

[233] Stanton AL, Ganz PA, Kwan L, et al. Outcomes from the Moving Beyond Cancer psychoeducational, randomized, controlled trial with breast cancer patients. *J. Clin. Oncol.* 2005 Sep 1;23(25):6009-18.

[234] Institute of Medicine. Cancer care for the whole patient: Meeting psychosocial needs. Washington, D.C., 2007.

[235] Akizuki N, Yamawaki S, Akechi T, Nakano T, Uchitomi Y. Development of an Impact Thermometer for use in combination with the Distress Thermometer as a brief screening tool for adjustment disorders and/or major depression in cancer patients. *J. Pain Symptom. Manage.* 2005 Jan;29(1):91-9.

[236] Gil F, Grassi L, Travado L, Tomamichel M, Gonzalez JR. Use of distress and depression thermometers to measure psychosocial morbidity among southern European cancer patients. *Supportive Care in Cancer.* 2005;13(8):600-6.

[237] Deck SM, Faul AC, Keeney C, Stone R, Studts JL. Predictors of Distress Thermometer ratings in breast cancer patients. 24th Annual Conference of the Association of Oncology Social Work. Louisville, KY: AOSW, 2008.

[238] Meyer MW, Mathew A, Naik LR. Psychosocial screening for distress. 24th Annual Conference of the Association of Oncology Social Work. Louisville, KY: AOSW, 2008.

[239] Rutland-Wallis M, Maddry H. Spirituality and faith: In dealth, spirituality can deepen meaning of life <http://www.athealth.com/Consumer/disorders/spirituality.html>. Accessed 2008 March 8, 2005.

[240] Stefanek M, McDonald PG, Hess SA. Religion, spirituality and cancer: Current status and methodological challenges. *Psycho-oncology.* 2004;14(6):450–63.

[241] Baldacchino D, Draper P. Spiritual coping strategies: a review of the nursing research literature. *Journal of advanced nursing.* 2001 Jun;34(6):833-41.

[242] Guglielmino JE. Cheryl Dudley: Inspired by faith, motivated by change <http://www.lbbc.org/content/newsletter-article/cheryl-dudley-inspired-by-faith-motivated-by-change.asp?section_tag=G>. Accessed 2008 March 8. *Living Beyond Breast Cancer,* 2005.

[243] Coughlin SS. Surviving cancer or other serious illness: a review of individual and community resources. CA: *a cancer journal for clinicians.* 2008 Jan-Feb;58(1):60-4.

[244] Jim HS, Richardson SA, Golden-Kreutz DM, Andersen BL. Strategies used in coping with a cancer diagnosis predict meaning in life for survivors. *Health Psychol.* 2006 Nov;25(6):753-61.

[245] Schneider MA. Broadening our perspective on spirituality and coping among women with breast cancer and their families: Implications for practice. *Indian Journal of Palliative Care.* 2007;13(2):25-31.

[246] Cancer Care Inc. Strengthening the spirit <http://www.cancercare.org/pdf/fact_sheets/fs_strength_spirit_en.pdf>. Accessed 2008 March 6. Cancer Care Inc., 2006.

[247] Kostiuk K. Spirituality Plays Important Role in Breast Cancer Information Processing for African-American Women. *Missouri School of Journalism* 2006 December.

[248] Gonnerman ME, Jr., Lutz GM, Yehieli M, Meisinger BK. Religion and health connection: a study of African American, protestant christians. *Journal of health care for the poor and underserved.* 2008 Feb;19(1):193-9.

[249] Loh KY. Handling spiritual questions of terminally ill patients. *Int. J. Palliat. Nurs.* 2004 Nov;10(11):550-1; discussion 2-3.

[250] Loh KY. Spiritual distress in a terminally ill patient with breast cancer. *Int. J. Palliat. Nurs.* 2004 Mar;10(3):131-2.

[251] Kim Y, Wellisch DK, Spillers RL, Crammer C. Psychological distress of female cancer caregivers: effects of type of cancer and caregivers' spirituality. *Support Care Cancer.* 2007 Dec;15(12):1367-74.

[252] Astrow AB, Wexler A, Texeira K, He MK, Sulmasy DP. Is failure to meet spiritual needs associated with cancer patients' perceptions of quality of care and their satisfaction with care? *J. Clin. Oncol.* 2007 Dec 20;25(36):5753-7.

[253] Crane-Okada R. A compass for the cancer journey: scientific, spiritual, and practical directives. *Oncology nursing forum.* 2007 Sep;34(5):945-55.

[254] NHMRC National Breast Cancer Centre Psychosocial Working Group. Psychosocial Clinical Practice Guidelines: Information, Support and Counselling for women with breast cancer. Sydney, Australia: National Health and Medical Research Council; 2000.

[255] Holland JC, Jacobsen PB, Riba MB. NCCN: Distress management. *Cancer Control.* 2001 Nov-Dec;8(6 Suppl 2):88-93.

[256] Johnson JD, Roberts CS, Cox CE, Reintgen DS, Levine JS, Parsons M. Breast cancer patients' personality style, age, and treatment decision making. *Journal of surgical oncology.* 1996 Nov;63(3):183-6.

[257] Blanchard CG, Labrecque MS, Ruckdeschel JC, Blanchard EB. Information and decision-making preferences of hospitalized adult cancer patients. *Soc. Sci. Med.* 1988;27(11):1139-45.

[258] Siminoff LA, Graham GC, Gordon NH. Cancer communication patterns and the influence of patient characteristics: disparities in information-giving and affective behaviors. *Patient education and counseling.* 2006 Sep;62(3):355-60.

[259] McWilliam CL, Brown JB, Stewart M. Breast cancer patients' experiences of patient-doctor communication: a working relationship. *Patient education and counseling.* 2000 Feb;39(2-3):191-204.

[260] Vitek L, Rosenzweig MQ, Stollings S. Distress in Patients With Cancer: Definition, Assessment, and Suggested Interventions. *Clinical Journal of Oncology Nursing.* 2007 06;11(3):413-8.

[261] Passik SD, Dugan W, McDonald MV, al. E. Oncologists' recognition of depression in their patients with cancer. *J. Clin. Oncol..* 1998;16:1594-600.

[262] Keller M, Sommerfeldt S, Fischer C, et al. Recognition of distress and psychiatric morbidity in cancer patients: a multi-method approach. *Ann. Oncol.* 2004 Aug; 15(8):1243-9.

[263] Ell K, Sanchez K, Vourlekis B, et al. Depression, correlates of depression, and receipt of depression care among low-income women with breast or gynecologic cancer. *J. Clin. Oncol.* 2005 May 1;23(13):3052-60.

[264] Ryan H, Schofield P, Cockburn J, et al. How to recognize and manage psychological distress in cancer patients. *European journal of cancer care.* 2005 Mar;14(1):7-15.

[265] Devine EC, Westlake SK. The effects of psychoeducational care provided to adults with cancer: meta-analysis of 116 studies. *Oncology nursing forum.* 1995 Oct;22(9):1369-81.

[266] McArdle JM, George WD, McArdle CS, et al. Psychological support for patients undergoing breast cancer surgery: a randomised study. *BMJ* (Clinical research ed. 1996 Mar 30;312(7034):813-6.

[267] Ganz PA, Polinsky ML, Schag CA, Heinrich RL. Rehabilitation of patients with primary breast cancer: assessing the impact of adjuvant therapy. *Recent Results Cancer Res.* 1989;115:244-54.

[268] Polinsky ML, Fred C, Ganz PA. Quantitative and qualitative assessment of a case management program for cancer patients. *Health and social work.* 1991 Aug;16(3):176-83.

[269] Ganz PA, Schag CC, Polinsky ML, Heinrich RL, Flack VF. Rehabilitation needs and breast cancer: the first month after primary therapy. *Breast Cancer Res. Treat.* 1987 Dec;10(3):243-53.

[270] Ganz PA, Coscarelli A, Fred C, Kahn B, Polinsky ML, Petersen L. Breast cancer survivors: psychosocial concerns and quality of life. *Breast Cancer Res. Treat.* 1996;38(2):183-99.

[271] Bowen DJ, Alfano CM, McGregor BA, et al. Possible socioeconomic and ethnic disparities in quality of life in a cohort of breast cancer survivors. *Breast Cancer Res. Treat.* 2007 Nov;106(1):85-95.

[272] Zebrack BJ, Yi J, Petersen L, Ganz PA. The impact of cancer and quality of life for long-term survivors. *Psycho-oncology.* 2007 Nov 29.

[273] Rehse B, Pukrop R. Effects of psychosocial interventions on quality of life in adult cancer patients: meta analysis of 37 published controlled outcome studies. *Patient education and counseling.* 2003 Jun;50(2):179-86.

[274] Scarvalone SA, Appling SE, Helzlsouer KJ, Oktay JS. Interdisciplinary Mind-Body Medicine Intervention for Breast Cancer Survivors: Social Work's Contribution. 24th Annual Conference of the Association of Oncology Social Work. Louisville, KY: AOSW, 2008.

[275] Saywell RM, Jr., Champion VL, Skinner CS, McQuillen D, Martin D, Maraj M. Cost-effectiveness comparison of five interventions to increase mammography screening. *Prev. Med.* 1999 Nov;29(5):374-82.

[276] Vogt TM, Glass A, Glasgow RE, La Chance PA, Lichtenstein E. The safety net: a cost-effective approach to improving breast and cervical cancer screening. *Journal of women's health* (2002). 2003 Oct;12(8):789-98.

[277] Lantz PM, Stencil D, Lippert MT, Beversdorf S, Jaros L, Remington PL. Breast and cervical cancer screening in a low-income managed care sample: the efficacy of physician letters and phone calls. *American journal of public health.* 1995 Jun;85(6):834-6.

[278] Marcus AC, Garrett KM, Cella D, et al. Telephone counseling of breast cancer patients after treatment: a description of a randomized clinical trial. *Psycho-oncology.* 1998 Nov-Dec;7(6):470-82.

[279] Moore ST. A social work practice model of case management: the case management grid. *Social work.* 1990 Sep;35(5):444-8.

[280] Weil M, Karls JM. Case Management in Human Service Practice. San Francisco: Jossey-Bass; 1985.

[281] Ussher J, Kirsten L, Butow P, Sandoval M. What do cancer support groups provide which other supportive relationships do not? The experience of peer support groups for people with cancer. *Soc. Sci. Med.* 2006 May;62(10):2565-76.

[282] Magen RH, Glajchen M. Cancer support groups: Client outcome and the context of group process. *Research on Social Work Practice.* 1999;9(5):541-54.

[283] Edelman S, Craig A, Kidman AD. Group intervention with cancer patients: Efficacy of psychoeducational versus supportive groups. *Journal of psychosocial oncology.* 2000;18(3):67-85.

[284] Newell SA, Sanson-Fisher RW, Savolainen NJ. Systematic review of psychological therapies for cancer patients: overview and recommendations for future research. *Journal of the National Cancer Institute.* 2002 Apr 17;94(8):558-84.

[285] Helgeson VS, Cohen S, Schulz R, Yasko J. Education and peer discussion group interventions and adjustment to breast cancer. *Arch. Gen. Psychiatry.* 1999 Apr;56(4):340-7.

[286] Monti DA, Peterson C, Kunkel EJ, et al. A randomized, controlled trial of mindfulness-based art therapy (MBAT) for women with cancer. Psycho-oncology. 2006 May;15(5):363-73.

[287] Bull J. Gilda's Club: *Philosophy and Progam.* New York, 1998.

[288] Rankin N, Williams P, Davis C, Girgis A. The use and acceptability of a one-on-one peer support program for Australian women with early breast cancer. *Patient education and counseling.* 2004 May;53(2):141-6.

[289] Davis C, Cohen RS, Apolinsky F. Providing social support to cancer patients: a look at alternative methods. *Journal of psychosocial oncology.* 2005;23(1):75-85.

[290] Klemm P, Bunnell D, Cullen M, et al. Online Cancer Support Groups: A Review of the Research Literature. CIN: *Computers, Informatics, Nursing.* 2003;21(3):136.

[291] Miller M. Onco chat: Online peer support for cancer survivors, families and friends <http://oncochat.org/>. Accessed 2008 April 30, 2007.

[292] Weinberg N. Online Help: Cancer Patients Participate in a Computer-Mediated Support Group. *Health and social work.* 1996;21(1):24-9.

[293] Klemm P, Hurst M, Dearholt SL, Trone SR. Gender differences on Internet cancer support groups. *Comput. Nurs.* 1999;17(2):65-72.

[294] Davis C, Williams P, Parle M, Redman S, Turner J. Assessing the support needs of women with early breast cancer in Australia. *Cancer nursing.* 2004 Mar-Apr;27(2):169-74.

[295] Northouse L, Kershaw T, Mood D, Schafenacker A. Effects of a family intervention on the quality of life of women with recurrent breast cancer and their family caregivers. *Psycho-oncology.* 2005;14(6):478-91.

[296] Hodgkinson K, Butow P, Hobbs KM, Wain G. After cancer: the unmet supportive care needs of survivors and their partners. *Journal of psychosocial oncology.* 2007;25(4):89-104.

[297] Mellon S, Northouse LL. Family survivorship and quality of life following a cancer diagnosis. *Research in Nursing and Health.* 2001;24(6):446-59.

[298] Northouse LL. Helping Families of Patients With Cancer. *Oncology nursing forum.* 2005;32(4):743-50.

[299] Northouse LL, Mood D, Kershaw T, et al. Quality of Life of Women With Recurrent Breast Cancer and Their Family Members. *Journal of Clinical Oncology.* 2002;20(19):4050.

[300] Northouse L, Templin T, Mood D. Couples'Adjustment to Breast Disease During the First Year Following Diagnosis. *Journal of Behavioral Medicine.* 2001;24(2):115-36.

[301] Williams P, Redman S, Rankin N, Davis C, Armstrong B, Malycha P. Is breast cancer care in accord with clinical practice guidelines: a consumer audit. *Breast* (Edinburgh, Scotland). 2002 Dec;11(6):509-15.

[302] National Cancer Institute. Facing forward: When someone you love has completed cancer treatment. Bethesda, MD: National Cancer Institute, 2005.

[303] Teixeira JF, Pletcher VM. Cancer Care Connection: An Innovative Approach Using Technology to "De-Frag" Access to Information, Community-Based Resources and Oncology Social Work Assessment and Coaching. 24th Annual Conference of the Association of Oncology Social Work. Louisville, KY: AOSW, 2008.

[304] Y-ME National Breast Cancer Organization. When the woman you love has breast cancer. Chicago, IL: *Y-ME National Breast Cancer Organization*, 2006.

[305] Bolte S. Sexuality, intimacy and cancer. *Life with Cancer* 2007.

[306] Cancer Care Inc. What can I say to a newly diagnosed loved one? New York, NY: Cancer Care Inc., 2007.

[307] Langhorne ME, Fulton JS, Otto SE. Oncology nursing. 5th ed. St. Louis, MO: Mosby Elsevier; 2007.

[308] Borstelmann NA, Cope RS. Current issues and ideas about men as caregivers. 24th Annual Conference of the Association of Oncology Social Work. Louisville, KY: AOSW, 2008.

[309] Carlson LE, Bultz BD, Speca M, St. Pierre M. Partners of cancer patients (Part II): Current psychosocial interventions and suggestions for improvement. *Journal of psychosocial oncology*. 2000;18(3):33-43.

[310] Christensen DN. Post mastectomy couple counseling: An outcome study of a structured treatment protocol. *Journal of Sex and Marital Therapy*. 1983;9(4):266-75.

[311] Gallo-Silver L. Sexual health awareness for people with cancer: An internet based response to commonly asked questions. 24th Annual Conference of the Association of Oncology Social Work. Louisville, KY: AOSW, 2008.

[312] Hodgkinson K, Butow P, Hunt GE, Wyse R, Hobbs KM, Wain G. Life after cancer: couples' and partners' psychological adjustment and supportive care needs. *Support Care Cancer*. 2007 Apr;15(4):405-15.

[313] Christ GH, Siegel K, Freund B, et al. Impact of parental terminal cancer on latency-age children. *Am. J. Orthopsychiatry*. 1993 Jul;63(3):417-25.

[314] American Cancer Society. Be honest with children about breast cancer <http://www.cancer.org/docroot/NWS/content/NWS_1_1x_Be_Honest_with_Children_About_Breast_Cancer.asp>. Accessed June 4, 2007, 2000.

[315] American Cancer Society. ACS: Be honest with your children about breast cancer <http://www.cancer.org/docroot/NWS/content/NWS_1_1x_Be_Honest_with_Children_About_Breast_Cancer.asp>. Accessed 2008 April 30, 2000.

[316] Rowland JH. Intrapersonal resources: Coping. In: Holland JC, Rowland JH (eds). Handbook of Psychooncology. New York: Oxford University Press, 1990:44-57.

[317] Logan-Carrillo C, Love G. The power of peer support: How to benefit from the wisdom of other survivors. In: Hoffman B (ed). A Cancer Survivor's Almanac. New York, NY: John Wiley, 2004:147-69.

[318] Zebrack B, Walsh-Burke K. Advocacy needs of adolescent and young adult cancer survivors: Perspectives of pediatric oncology social workers. *Journal of psychosocial oncology*. 2004;22(2):75-87.

[319] National Coalition for Cancer Survivorship. NCCS National Coalition for Cancer Survivorship <http://canceradvocacy.org/>. Accessed 2008 April 30, 2008.

[320] Fawcett SB, Paine-Andrews A, Francisco VT, et al. Using empowerment theory in collaborative partnerships for community health and development. *Am. J. Community Psychol.* 1995 Oct;23(5):677-97.

[321] Bastian H. Speaking up for ourselves - The evolution of consumer advocacy in health care. *International Journal of Technology Assessment in Health Care.* 1998;14:3-23.

[322] McCabe MS, Varricchio CG, Padberg R, Simpson N. Women's health advocacy: Its growth and development in oncology. *Seminars in oncology nursing.* 1994;11:137-42.

[323] Gillette J. Advocacy and nursing: Implications for women's health care. Australian *Journal of Advanced Nursing.* 1998;6:4-11.

[324] Davis C, Salo L, Redman S. Evaluating the effectiveness of advocacy training for breast cancer advocates in Australia. *European journal of cancer care.* 2001 Jun;10(2):82-6.

[325] Liberati A. Consumer participation in research and health care. *British Medical Journal.* 1997 Aug 30;315(7107):499.

[326] Batt S. The Politics of Breast Cancer. Melbourne, Australia: Spinifex Press; 1996.

[327] Datloff EH. The international politics of breast cancer: The power of advocacy. *Helix Amgen's Magazine of Biotechnology.* 1997;3:42-7.

[328] Muha L. The redefinition of patient advocacy - Pillars of strength. Odyssey. 1997;3:2-7.

[329] National Breast Cancer Coalition (NBCC). NBCC <http://www.stopbreastcancer.org/index.php>. Accessed 2008 April 30, 2008.

[330] National Breast Cancer Coalition. Leadership, Education and Advocacy Development. Washington, DC, 1998.

[331] Cancer Care Inc. About us <http://www.cancercare.org/about_us/>. Accessed 2008 April 30, n.d.

[332] American Association for Cancer Research (AACR). About us <http://www.aacr.org/home/about-us.aspx>. Accessed 2008 April 30, 2008.

[333] Swarz JA, Ellis SF, Ousley A, Walsh KE, Zebrack B. Evidence-Based Practice in Oncology Social Work: Selected Findings from the National Practitioner Information Needs Analysis Study. 24th Annual Conference of the Association of Oncology Social Work. Louisville, KY: AOSW, 2008.

[334] Collaboration C. The Cochrane Collaboration: The reliable source of information in health care <http://www.cochrane.org/>. Accessed 2008 June 27. Cochrane Collaboration, Oxford, England, 2008.

[335] Davis C. Hospital social work: Are we conducting the right type of research? *Social work in health care.* 2004;38(3):67-9.

[336] Rizzo VM, Abrams A. Utilization review: A powerful social work role in health care settings. *Health and Social Work.* 2000;25(4):264-9.

[337] Cowles LA, Lefcowitz MJ. Interdisciplinary expectations of the medical social worker in the hospital setting: Part 2. *Health and Social Work.* 1995;20:279-87.

[338] Egan M, Kadushin G. Rural hospital social work: Views of physicians and social workers. *Social work in health care.* 1997;26:1-21.

INDEX

A

abusive, 36
accommodation, 30, 116
accountability, 38, 93
accounting, 10, 46
acculturation, 26
ACE, 34, 116
acute, 41, 57, 69, 74, 76, 78
adaptation, 70, 118
adjustment, 21, 33, 52, 55, 61, 73, 107, 118, 119, 120, 123, 124
administration, 2, 38, 110
adult, 69, 121, 122, 124
adults, 15, 44, 104, 121
advocacy, 1, 2, 6, 7, 34, 69, 72, 81, 82, 83, 84, 88, 89, 91, 107, 119, 125
affiliates, 89
Africa, 13
African American, 5, 11, 12, 23, 24, 25, 27, 28, 62, 108, 111, 112, 113, 119, 120
African American women, 5, 11, 12, 23, 24, 25, 28, 112, 113, 119
African Americans, 11, 12, 24, 111
African-American, 52, 112, 113, 120
age, 9, 15, 16, 17, 18, 22, 23, 24, 40, 45, 52, 67, 74, 79, 88, 111, 112, 117, 119, 121, 124
agent, 77
agents, 13
aging, 15
agricultural, 35
aid, 71
AIDS, 19, 25, 83
Alaska, 11, 12, 25, 27, 114
Alaska Natives, 25, 27, 114
alcohol, 14, 15
alcohol consumption, 15
alcohol use, 14

alternative, 46, 68, 69, 87, 123
ambiguity, 33
amendments, 88
American Cancer Society (ACS), 5, 10, 43, 50, 58, 65, 80, 88, 100, 102, 103, 109, 110, 111, 113, 124
American Indian, 11, 12, 24, 25, 27, 113, 114
American Psychological Association, 119
analgesics, 52
anger, 32, 66, 75
animals, 14
antidepressant, 29
antidepressant medication, 29
antidepressants, 68
ants, 53, 59
anxiety, 21, 33, 61, 68, 69, 70, 77, 78, 79
APA, 37
Appalachia, 29, 114
applied research, 5
Arizona, 113
Asia, 13
Asian, 11, 12, 25, 27, 28, 114
Asian American, 25, 27, 28, 114
Asian Americans, 25, 27, 114
assessment, 2, 7, 46, 53, 58, 66, 115, 122
assumptions, 25
attitudes, 25, 68, 112, 113
atypical, 75
Australia, 13, 65, 67, 84, 119, 121, 123, 125
autonomy, 39
availability, 13, 30, 62
avoidant, 61
awareness, 70, 77, 124

B

babies, 20, 79
bankruptcy, 40, 45
barrier, 29, 44, 56, 72

barriers, 3, 5, 6, 7, 23, 25, 26, 28, 37, 40, 43, 44, 68, 82, 96, 112
behavior, 108, 112, 114
belief systems, 63
beliefs, 13, 23, 25, 26, 28, 59, 60, 62, 63, 68, 112, 114
benefits, 19, 31, 39, 40, 56, 60, 61, 67, 68, 70, 94, 116
benign, 118
bereavement, 2
betrayal, 75
beverages, 15
biopsy, 6, 12, 109, 118
birth, 10, 18
black women, 11
blaming, 32
bleeding, 77
blood, 18, 61
blood clot, 18
blood pressure, 61
blurring, 95
body image, 23, 52, 77
Boston, 108
breast cancer, 5, 9, 10, 11, 12, 13, 14, 15, 16, 17, 18, 19, 20, 21, 23, 24, 25, 26, 27, 29, 30, 41, 45, 46, 52, 55, 56, 65, 67, 68, 69, 71, 74, 76, 78, 83, 84, 85, 87, 88, 89, 107, 109, 110, 111, 112, 113, 114, 115, 116, 117, 118, 119, 120, 121, 122, 123, 124, 125
breast carcinoma, 111, 117, 118
breast feeding, 17
breathing, 58
Bronx, 108
Brussels, 84
building blocks, 4

C

Canada, 43, 84
cancer care, 1, 2, 4, 6, 14, 45, 56, 68, 82, 84, 88, 89, 96, 110, 116, 119, 121, 124, 125
cancer cells, 11, 31
cancer screening, 25, 28, 43, 44, 108, 112, 113
cancer treatment, 1, 2, 3, 12, 22, 28, 29, 30, 31, 32, 52, 53, 56, 57, 58, 59, 61, 69, 74, 77, 78, 88, 110, 114, 115, 117, 119, 124
capacity, 82
carcinoma, 111, 117, 118
care model, 41, 57
caregiver, ix, 46, 53, 63, 74, 75
caregivers, 1, 2, 47, 62, 63, 76, 91, 115, 121, 123, 124
caretaker, 31
Catholic, 62

Caucasian, 11, 12, 23, 52, 62
CDC, 5, 108, 109
cell, 17
Census Bureau, 109, 113
Central America, 13
cervical cancer, 10, 12, 13, 14, 15, 16, 17, 18, 19, 24, 27, 29, 109, 110, 113, 114, 122
cervix, 10, 26, 112
CES, 37
charities, 6
check-ups, 31
chemotherapy, 14, 22, 24, 29, 30, 45, 49, 66, 76, 77, 79, 118
childcare, 21, 23, 30, 47, 49, 50, 58
childrearing, 50
children, v, ix, 2, 22, 30, 49, 50, 55, 58, 62, 67, 68, 75, 76, 78, 79, 80, 93, 105, 124
chlamydia, 19
chronic disease, 74
chronic illness, 40, 41
CIN, 123
citizens, 36, 37, 43, 97
classes, 71
classification, 27
cleaning, 30
clients, 7, 25, 70, 83, 94
clinical trial, 6, 84, 89, 91, 94, 122
clinical trials, 6, 84, 89, 91, 94
clinically significant, 119
clinician, 68
clinics, 52, 71, 91
Cochrane, 91, 125
cognitive, 69
cognitive-behavioral therapies, 69
cohesion, 70
cohort, 45, 116, 122
Cold War, 37
collaboration, 82, 94
Collaboration, 91, 125
colon, 16, 110, 115
colon cancer, 16, 110
Colorado, 37
colorectal cancer, 16, 43
common symptoms, 18
communication, 5, 7, 28, 30, 33, 53, 56, 65, 72, 75, 76, 81, 116, 121
communication skills, 56
communism, 37
communities, ix, 2, 6, 7, 25, 26, 31, 71, 72, 89, 112
community, 2, 5, 6, 24, 26, 52, 59, 60, 62, 69, 70, 71, 81, 82, 84, 89, 91, 97, 108, 113, 120, 125
compensation, 36, 37, 39
competency, 81

competition, 37
compliance, 4, 55
complications, 9, 18
components, 6, 82, 87, 118
composition, 60
concentration, 58
conception, 22
conflict, 61
congruence, 24
consciousness, 25
consensus, 60
constipation, 58
constraints, 41
consultants, 116
consumerism, 40
consumers, 39, 40, 83, 84, 87
consumption, 15
continuity, 39, 96
contraceptives, 17, 18
control, 3, 32, 38, 39, 54, 61, 69, 70, 109, 112, 119
controlled studies, 69
controlled trials, 69
cookies, 104
cooking, 72
copayment, 44
coping, 90, 115, 118, 124
coping strategies, 4, 33, 72, 75, 81, 120
coping strategy, 61
correlation, 14, 45
cost analyses, 47
cost-effective, 7, 69, 70, 93, 94, 122
costs, 32, 38, 39, 40, 41, 43, 44, 46, 47, 95
counsel, 2
counseling, 2, 20, 31, 66, 67, 68, 69, 72, 76, 77, 79, 80, 88, 95, 108, 109, 121, 122, 123, 124
country of origin, 26
couples, 124
coverage, 12, 37, 40, 41, 43, 44, 45, 46, 117
crying, 76
cultural beliefs, 13, 23
cultural differences, 13
cultural factors, 111
culture, 14, 25, 26, 28, 35, 110
curing, 68

D

dairy, 14
Dallas, 36
data collection, 27
database, 87, 94
dating, 22
death, 10, 11, 12, 13, 15, 16, 26, 27, 29, 32, 47, 71
death rate, 10, 11, 12, 26, 29

deaths, 9, 10, 11, 13, 16, 24, 27
decision making, 31, 55, 76, 119, 121
decision-making process, 56
decisions, 26, 28, 29, 31, 33, 52, 53, 54, 56, 61, 64, 70, 72, 76, 82, 83, 87, 97, 116
deductibles, 39
defense, 43
definition, 6, 44, 59
delivery, 5, 7, 18, 38, 39, 97
democracy, 37
demographic factors, 44
denial, 75
Department of Defense, 83
Department of Health and Human Services, 113, 117
depressed, 53, 66, 67, 68
depression, 21, 23, 26, 29, 53, 58, 61, 69, 77, 107, 115, 120, 121
depressive disorder, 69
detection, 6, 11, 24, 26, 44, 56, 65, 96, 109
developed countries, 13
developing countries, 13
diabetes, 14, 85
diarrhea, 58
diet, 13, 14, 26, 27, 89
dietary, 13
dietary habits, 13
diets, 14, 26
directives, 121
disability, 20, 37, 46, 47, 51
disclosure, 78, 116
discomfort, 28, 77
discrimination, 25
discs, 82
diseases, 19
dissatisfaction, 40
disseminate, 88
distress, 22, 55, 56, 57, 58, 59, 61, 62, 63, 65, 68, 69, 70, 72, 96, 107, 108, 118, 119, 120, 121
diversity, 6, 26, 27
divorce, 75
DNA, 16, 17, 19
DNA damage, 17
doctors, 5, 21, 22, 23, 24, 26, 30, 31, 33, 34, 35, 41, 51, 52, 57, 76, 107, 116
dominance, 40
drugs, 17, 34
duration, 52, 69, 70
duties, 6, 7, 49
dysplasia, 114

E

ears, 22
eating, 58

economic status, 44
education, 34, 84, 108, 116, 123, 125
educational programs, 27, 84, 88, 91
educational services, 88
educators, 3
elderly, 19, 37, 38, 40
emotional, v, ix, 2, 3, 21, 28, 29, 31, 52, 53, 55, 59, 61, 65, 66, 68, 71, 73, 75, 77, 78, 79, 89, 96
emotional distress, 53, 65, 68, 71, 78, 96
emotional health, 79
emotional reactions, 79
emotional state, 28
emotional well-being, 3
emotions, 31, 32, 57, 66, 75, 78, 79
empathy, 70
employees, 36, 37, 38, 40, 95
employers, 36, 37, 38, 39, 40, 41, 82
employment, 21, 29, 30, 37, 40, 44, 51, 53
employment status, 29
empowered, 65, 66
empowerment, 3, 7, 61, 70, 72, 81, 82, 108, 125
endocrine, 68
end-of-life care, 34
endometrial cancer, 11, 12, 14, 16, 18, 19, 26, 110
endometriosis, 17
energy, 19, 53, 70, 77, 79
England, 125
enrollment, 6, 38, 39
environment, 35, 63, 71, 82, 89
environmental effects, 13
environmental protection, 35
epidemiology, 84, 110
equality, 37
estimating, 33
estrogen, 15, 18, 19, 22
estrogens, 17
ethnic groups, 11, 12, 13, 27, 111, 112
ethnic minority, 25, 26, 27, 44, 112
ethnicity, 9, 44, 109, 110, 111, 113
Europe, 14
evidence-based practices, 90
evolution, 35, 125
exercise, 15, 20, 26
expenditures, 43, 46, 47, 117
expertise, 41, 105
exposure, 13, 18, 19
eye contact, 28

family, ix, 1, 2, 4, 5, 11, 16, 17, 20, 22, 23, 24, 25, 26, 28, 30, 31, 32, 34, 35, 40, 43, 44, 47, 49, 50, 51, 52, 53, 56, 60, 61, 62, 63, 66, 67, 69, 70, 71, 72, 73, 74, 75, 78, 79, 80, 81, 82, 84, 94, 105, 111, 116, 123
family history, 16, 17
family income, 43, 44
family life, 30
family members, 31, 47, 50, 62, 63, 71, 74, 75, 78, 82, 94, 111
family system, 79
fat, 14, 26
fatalistic, 61
fatigue, 52, 53, 58, 61, 77, 78
fats, 14
fear, 31, 32, 34, 37, 57, 62, 68, 75, 79, 115
fears, 30, 58, 70, 76, 77, 78
federal government, 37, 38, 39, 41, 95
federal law, 51
feeding, 17
feelings, 26, 28, 30, 50, 59, 62, 68, 69, 70, 74, 75, 78, 79
femininity, ix, 22, 52
feminist, 115
fertility, 17, 22
Filipino, 28, 114
financial barriers, 37
financial difficulty, 45
financial distress, 55
financial instability, 46
financing, 38, 117
focus group, 30
focusing, 3, 57
food, 44
Food and Drug Administration, 19
forecasting, 34
formal education, 1, 82
framing, 57
France, 43
Franklin D. Roosevelt, 37
freedom, 59
friendship, 71
fruits, 14
frustration, 65
funding, 5, 83, 94
fundraising, 84, 85

F

failure, 40, 121
faith, 60, 62, 63, 120
familial, 35, 116

G

GDP, 43
gender, 9, 31, 45, 108, 115
genes, 16
genetic testing, 17, 20
genetics, 9, 16, 41

Germany, 43
goal setting, 72, 82
goals, 2, 34, 89
God, 20, 22, 25, 32, 59, 60, 61, 62, 63
gonorrhea, 19
Gore, 118
gossip, 30
government, 6, 36, 37, 39, 41, 95
grants, 88, 94
grassroots, 83, 84
Great Depression, 37
grief, 55
gross domestic product, 43
group therapy, 69
group work, 81
groups, 5, 6, 11, 12, 13, 14, 24, 25, 26, 27, 28, 29,
    38, 39, 44, 70, 71, 72, 76, 78, 79, 84, 85, 111,
    112, 122, 123
growth, 17, 22, 38, 39, 125
guidance, 33
guidelines, 65, 87, 88, 124
guilt, 32, 49, 75
guilty, 32, 37, 78
gynecological cancers, 10, 18, 110, 121

H

hair loss, 79
hands, 20, 61
hardships, 43
Harlem, 112
hate, 32, 50, 66
headache, 32
healing, 26, 119
health, ix, 1, 2, 3, 4, 5, 6, 7, 9, 13, 14, 20, 21, 22, 23,
    24, 25, 26, 27, 28, 29, 30, 34, 35, 36, 37, 38, 39,
    40, 41, 43, 44, 45, 46, 47, 49, 52, 53, 54, 55, 56,
    61, 63, 65, 66, 68, 71, 72, 75, 77, 81, 82, 83, 84,
    87, 88, 89, 91, 93, 94, 95, 97, 108, 109,
    110, 111, 112, 113, 114, 115, 116, 117, 119,
    120, 122, 124, 125
Health and Human Services (HHS), 5, 108, 117
health care, 1, 2, 3, 4, 5, 6, 7, 13, 14, 24, 26, 28, 34,
    35, 36, 37, 38, 39, 40, 41, 43, 44, 46, 47, 52, 53,
    54, 56, 65, 66, 68, 71, 72, 77, 82, 83, 84, 87, 88,
    91, 93, 94, 95, 97, 112, 117, 119, 120, 125
health care costs, 40, 43, 44, 46, 95
health care professionals, 3, 34, 66, 71, 84, 88, 94
health care system, 2, 3, 5, 6, 14, 35, 37, 38, 41, 56,
    72, 83, 93, 94, 97
health education, 2
health insurance, 6, 14, 20, 23, 37, 38, 40, 41, 43, 45,
    46, 47, 49, 113, 117
health locus of control, 112

health problems, 2
health services, 29, 30, 37, 44
health status, 30, 36, 55, 117
healthcare, 39, 41
hearing, 32, 67
heart, 15, 85
heart disease, 15, 85
Helix, 125
helplessness, 61
herbal, 26
herbal therapy, 26
high risk, 16, 17, 67
high-fat, 14
high-risk, 19
hip, 65
Hispanic, 11, 12, 24, 25, 26, 27, 28, 62, 100, 112,
    113, 114
Hispanic population, 12, 112, 113
Hispanics, 12, 24, 25, 52, 113
HMOs, 36, 38, 39, 40
holistic, ix, 4, 64, 69
holistic approach, 69
Holland, 119, 121, 124
homeless, 43, 46, 47
honesty, 75, 79
honey, 74, 85
hormone, 16, 18, 77
hormones, 15, 17
hospice, 6, 33, 34, 91
hospital, 24, 28, 36, 38, 39, 46, 68, 81, 94, 95, 96,
    118, 125
hospital care, 36
hospitalized, 121
hospitals, 1, 35, 36, 37, 38, 39, 40, 71, 91, 97
host, 57
household, 30, 40, 44, 46, 47, 75, 79
household income, 40, 44, 46
housing, 36, 46, 58
human, 10, 19, 110
human immunodeficiency virus (HIV/AIDS), 19, 85
human papilloma virus (HPV), 10, 15, 18, 19, 110
husband, 2, 22, 49, 56, 63, 73, 74, 75, 76, 77, 79, 82,
    84, 105
hypnosis, 72
hysterectomy, 17

I

identification, 27
ideology, 37
imagery, 71
immigrants, 35
immune function, 61
immune system, 18, 19

in transition, 107
in utero, 18
incidence, 9, 11, 12, 13, 14, 15, 18, 21, 23, 24, 26,
    27, 114
income, 13, 23, 24, 29, 40, 41, 43, 44, 45, 46, 47, 52,
    68, 108, 112, 114, 121, 122
incomes, 29
increased access, 38
incurable, 34, 116
independence, 74
Indian, 12, 27, 120
Indians, 25, 27
indication, 31
industrialization, 35
industrialized countries, 13, 43
industry, 36, 38
inefficiency, 37
inequality, 7
infection, 10, 18, 19
infections, 19
infertile, 17
infertility, 17, 22
inflation, 40
infrastructure, 5, 35, 37
inherited, 16
injuries, 37
injustice, 110
insecurity, 37
inspiration, ix
insurance, 6, 7, 12, 14, 20, 23, 35, 36, 37, 38, 39, 40,
    41, 43, 44, 45, 46, 47, 49, 51, 58, 75, 81, 82, 93,
    110, 117
insurance companies, 39, 41, 75, 81, 82
integration, 109
interactions, 26, 28, 30, 33
interdependence, 74
interdisciplinary, 4
internal organization, 3, 70
internet, 72, 76, 77, 87, 124
Internet, 87, 89, 123
interpersonal relations, 65
interpretation, 51
interrelationships, 115
interval, 45
intervention, 21, 23, 69, 70, 93, 94, 118, 123
intimacy, 77, 124
invasive, 9, 11, 29, 45
invasive cancer, 11
investment, 36
irritation, 77
isolation, 26, 30, 55, 70

J

JAMA, 110, 116, 117
Japan, 13, 14
Japanese, 13, 27
jobs, 29, 37, 51
Jun, 111, 112, 114, 115, 117, 118, 120, 122, 125
jurisdictions, 33
justice, 37

K

Kaiser Family Foundation, 40, 116, 117
Korean, 27

L

labor, 35, 36
language, 25, 26, 31, 56, 96
language barrier, 26, 96
Laotian, 27
large-scale, 94
latency, 124
late-stage, 111
Latino, 113
Latinos, 112, 113
law, 6, 36
laws, 41, 51
leadership, 34, 84
learning, 32, 70, 75, 82
legislation, 36
lending, 4
life expectancy, 31, 33, 34
lifestyle, 16, 26, 27
lifetime, 9, 11, 17
likelihood, 19, 75
limitations, 51, 57
links, 73, 87, 88, 89, 91
listening, 56, 69, 76
literacy, 23, 68
living conditions, 13, 14
lobby, 41, 89
location, 60, 71
long distance, 30, 51
long period, 17, 29, 50
loss of control, 61
love, 53, 74, 91, 124
low-income, 14, 23, 24, 29, 40, 41, 45, 47, 52, 68,
    108, 112, 114, 121, 122
lymphoma, 118

M

major depression, 68, 120

maladaptive, 55, 56
malignancy, 9, 10, 29
malignant, 17
mammogram, 6, 13, 21, 23, 24, 25, 45, 112
mammography, 29, 43, 112, 122
management, 2, 7, 32, 39, 54, 56, 65, 69, 89, 107, 109, 115, 121, 122
mandates, 88
market, 38, 40
marriage, 23, 77
Massachusetts, 41, 117
mastectomy, 22, 23, 24, 29, 52, 124
meals, 60
meat, 14
media, 88
median, 15, 16
Medicaid, 14, 39, 40, 45
medical care, 1, 14, 24, 30, 35, 36, 37, 44, 45, 74, 82, 95
medical services, 36, 38, 46
medically underserved populations, 81
Medicare, 39, 40, 45
medication, 52, 68, 77, 118
medications, 29, 46, 49, 66
medicine, 26, 35, 38, 39, 41, 87, 108, 115, 116, 117, 119
meditation, 60
Medline, 87
melanoma, 10
membership, 91
memory, 22, 58
men, 3, 16, 45, 70, 72, 75, 76, 88, 108, 124
menopause, 15, 17, 18, 21, 22, 77
menstruation, 17, 78
mental health, 29, 30, 68
meta analysis, 122
meta-analysis, 69, 118, 121
metabolic, 68
metastatic, 33, 34, 115, 116
metastatic cancer, 34
metastatic disease, 33, 115
Mexico, 113
middle class, 38
midlife, 15
migrant, 112
migration, 13
Mind-Body, 122
minorities, 40, 44
minority, 1, 5, 12, 25, 26, 27, 34, 44, 45, 46, 47, 52, 53, 95, 112
minority groups, 25
mirror, 55
miscarriage, 17

misconceptions, 114
misleading, 87
Missouri, 120
misunderstanding, 33
modalities, 31, 56
models, 3, 38, 56, 57, 96, 97
money, 41, 44, 45, 46
mood, 21, 22, 67, 69, 118
mood disorder, 118
mood swings, 22
morbidity, 74, 107, 118, 120, 121
morning, 53
mortality, 5, 10, 11, 12, 13, 21, 23, 26, 27, 47, 63, 75, 110, 111, 112, 114
mortality rate, 5, 11, 12, 13, 21, 23, 26, 27, 47
mothers, 18, 22, 49, 50
motion, 17
mouth, 58, 78
movement, ix, 7, 36, 38, 83
MSW, 2
multidisciplinary, 1, 2, 82
multimedia, 89
muscles, 11
music, 60, 71
mutations, 16
mutuality, 70

N

nation, 5, 35, 36, 37, 38, 41, 43, 89
National Research Council, 107
nausea, 58, 69, 77, 78
negative consequences, 95
neglect, 28
negotiating, 39
negotiation, 81
nervousness, 58
Netherlands, 13
network, 83, 84
networking, 71, 91
New England, 117, 119
New Mexico, 113
New York, 108, 116, 119, 123, 124
New Zealand, 115
next generation, 18
Nixon, 38
non-clinical, 71
non-English speaking, 114
non-profit, 38
non-smokers, 15
normal, 19, 29, 49, 50, 53, 57, 66, 68, 76, 78, 79
norms, 52
not-for-profit, 91
nurse, 2, 76, 95, 119

Nurse practitioners, 3
nurses, 1, 4, 6, 57, 82, 95, 117
nursing, 107, 111, 112, 114, 120, 121, 123, 124, 125

O

obese, 14
obesity, 14
obligation, 36
obligations, 30
Odyssey, 125
Office of Management and Budget (OMB), 40
Oklahoma, 36
online, 72, 89, 90, 91
on-line, 82
openness, 79
optimism, 118
oral, 17, 18
oral contraceptives, 17, 18
organ, 10
organization, 39, 81, 84, 89, 91
organizations, 1, 3, 6, 39, 71, 78, 82, 83, 90, 91
out-of-pocket, 40, 43, 44, 46, 47, 49, 117
outpatient, 91
outpatients, 107
ovarian cancer, 9, 10, 14, 15, 16, 17, 19, 29, 63, 84, 89, 109
ovarian cancers, 10, 16, 29
ovarian tumor, 17
ovaries, 9, 18
ovary, 10, 109
overload, 56, 90
oversight, 36
over-the-counter, 49
overweight, 14
ovulation, 15, 17

P

Pacific, 11, 12, 25, 26, 27, 114
Pacific Islander, 11, 12, 25, 26, 27, 114
packets, 84
pain, 25, 31, 52, 53, 58, 61, 69, 77, 78, 79
palliative, 24, 34
palliative care, 24, 34
Pap, 10, 13, 29
parents, 16, 53, 79, 80
Parkinson, 104
partnership, 3
partnerships, 6, 94, 125
passive, 28, 61
patients, ix, 1, 2, 3, 4, 5, 6, 24, 26, 28, 29, 30, 31, 33, 34, 43, 46, 51, 52, 55, 56, 62, 63, 65, 68, 69, 71, 75, 81, 82, 83, 88, 91, 93, 94, 107, 108, 110, 111,
113, 114, 115, 116, 117, 118, 119, 120, 121, 122, 123, 124
pediatric, 124
peer, 70, 71, 72, 82, 83, 90, 108, 122, 123, 124
peer review, 83
peer support, 71, 82, 122, 123, 124
pelvic, 19
Pennsylvania, 89
perceptions, 36, 107, 111, 115, 121
periodic, 70
personal, ix, 20, 28, 40, 52, 60, 62, 63, 65, 71, 72, 73, 82, 110
personal control, 40
personal life, 62
personal relationship, 62, 63
personality, 121
philosophy, 39, 59
phone, 33, 122
physical activity, 15, 26, 89
physical exercise, 15
physical health, 61, 70
physical well-being, 3
physicians, 1, 2, 4, 29, 30, 33, 34, 35, 36, 37, 38, 39, 58, 63, 65, 82, 88, 115, 116, 125
Physicians, 38, 77, 113
physiological, 61
planning, 7, 54, 76
play, ix, 1, 3, 13, 16, 17, 23, 28, 37, 50, 51, 52, 63, 66, 80, 82, 93
policy makers, 41, 84
political stability, 37
politics, 125
polyunsaturated fat, 14
poor, 13, 30, 31, 33, 34, 36, 38, 40, 44, 55, 56, 67, 72, 73, 112, 117, 120
population, 12, 18, 21, 24, 26, 27, 29, 36, 38, 41, 43, 44, 49, 74, 97, 111, 113, 117
population group, 24, 44
positive behaviors, 3
poverty, 13, 14, 24, 26, 29, 37, 117
power, 53, 60, 61, 62, 63, 119, 124, 125
powers, 54
predictors, 12
pre-existing, 2, 41
pregnancy, 17, 18, 21, 22, 111
pregnant, 18, 22
premium, 39
premiums, 40, 43, 49
president, 36, 37
President Bush, 6
pressure, 61, 90
prevention, 2, 6, 37, 44, 56, 89, 96, 109, 110, 112, 113

preventive, 24, 25, 29, 38
primary care, 39, 112
privacy, 25, 30, 72
private, 12, 14, 39, 40, 41, 43, 44, 45, 46
probability, 15
probe, 4, 68
problem solving, 72, 81, 82
problem-solving, 111
production, 35
productivity, 43
professional development, 91
professions, 1
profit, 38, 39, 91
progesterone, 18, 19, 22
prognosis, 31, 33, 34, 79, 111, 115, 116
program, 6, 14, 24, 37, 43, 44, 45, 46, 84, 88, 89,
    117, 122, 123
proliferation, 17
promote, 37, 69
prosperity, 38
prostate cancer, 108
prostheses, 49
protection, 15, 35, 51
protective factors, 26
protocol, 124
provider networks, 39
psychiatric illness, 66
psychiatric morbidity, 118, 121
psychoeducational intervention, 70
psychological distress, 21, 59, 63, 66, 70, 74, 118,
    119, 121
psychological problems, 68
psychological variables, 113
psychological well-being, 57, 68
psychologist, 66
psychosocial functioning, 2
psychosocial support, 66, 70
psychotherapy, 69, 118
public, 12, 37, 39, 40, 44, 45, 50, 51, 65, 85, 88, 89,
    90, 108, 111, 113, 114, 115, 116, 122
public education, 85
public health, 37, 40, 65, 108, 111, 113, 114, 115,
    116, 122

Q

quality of life (QOL), 1, 2, 3, 4, 21, 24, 29, 33, 34,
    53, 61, 65, 68, 69, 77, 93, 107, 111, 114, 118,
    122, 123

R

race, 9, 12, 14, 44, 88, 109, 110, 111, 113
racial differences, 111

racial groups, 27
radiation, 14, 19, 22, 24, 29, 30, 41, 45, 77, 115
radiation therapy, 14, 19, 22, 29, 45, 77, 115
range, 2, 34, 69, 74, 75, 77, 79, 89
ratings, 120
realism, 116
reality, 60
receptors, 16
recognition, 28, 68, 107, 121
reconstruction, 23, 52
reconstructive surgery, 45
recovery, 52
recreational, 71
rectum, 115
recurrence, 31, 32, 33, 67, 70, 111, 115
red meat, 14
reduction, 17, 111
reflection, 119
reforms, 36
regional, 107, 113
registries, 110
registry, 45
regular, 10, 13, 23, 24, 26, 28, 29
regulations, 36
rehabilitation, 69
reimbursement, 38, 39
relationship, 14, 15, 17, 19, 40, 59, 61, 62, 65, 69,
    75, 76, 78, 116, 121
relationships, 30, 39, 60, 63, 67, 74, 75, 77, 119, 122
relatives, 16
relaxation, 69, 71, 72
reliability, 87
religion, 59, 60, 62, 63
religiosity, 59
religious belief, 26, 59, 60, 62
religious beliefs, 26, 59, 60
remission, 57
rent, 49
research, ix, 2, 5, 6, 10, 14, 15, 16, 17, 18, 19, 21, 24,
    25, 37, 38, 46, 47, 57, 61, 63, 70, 71, 72, 81, 82,
    83, 84, 85, 88, 89, 90, 91, 93, 94, 112, 113, 116,
    119, 120, 121, 123, 125
researchers, 9, 10, 12, 13, 14, 16, 17, 18, 33, 46, 57,
    59, 63, 84, 88, 94
resilience, 115
resistance, 96
resources, 1, 2, 4, 5, 7, 11, 14, 20, 24, 28, 41, 51, 62,
    63, 69, 70, 78, 80, 82, 83, 84, 87, 88, 89, 95, 120,
    124
responsibilities, 7, 22, 49, 50, 61, 79, 88
restructuring, 95
retirement, 47
revenue, 95

Reynolds, 108
Rhode Island, 45
risk, 9, 11, 12, 13, 14, 15, 16, 17, 18, 19, 20, 21, 24, 26, 38, 39, 40, 44, 45, 47, 55, 63, 67, 69, 70, 95, 110, 111, 113, 116, 118
risk assessment, 70
risk behaviors, 14
risk factors, 13, 15, 16, 17, 19, 20, 26, 110
risk perception, 113
risks, 20, 24, 31, 39, 56
role conflict, 95
routines, 26, 49
rural, 28, 29, 30, 35, 36, 38, 40, 51, 62, 70, 72, 114, 115
rural areas, 29, 72
rural communities, 30, 62
rural population, 29
rural women, 29, 30, 51, 114, 115

S

sadness, 22, 55, 58
safeguard, 37
safety, 36, 122
salary, 40
sample, 30, 60, 90, 115, 118, 122
satisfaction, 4, 6, 28, 63, 77, 115, 121
saturated fat, 14
savings, 43, 47, 93
scarcity, 25
school, 2, 36, 53, 58, 79
scientists, 15, 84, 119
screening programs, 11, 13
search, 90, 91
searching, 25
secret, 25
security, 2
self, 83, 99, 107
self worth, 93
self-care, 69, 79, 114
self-efficacy, 108
self-esteem, 77
self-report, 29, 46, 61
separation, 75
service provider, 68
services, 1, 2, 3, 4, 5, 6, 7, 13, 24, 25, 29, 30, 34, 35, 37, 38, 39, 40, 41, 44, 56, 66, 68, 70, 72, 74, 75, 78, 81, 82, 83, 84, 87, 88, 96, 97, 109
settlements, 36
sex, 19, 67, 77
sexual activity, 28
sexual contact, 18
sexual health, 77
sexuality, ix, 77

sexually transmitted disease, 19
sexually transmitted diseases, 19
shares, 36
sharing, 71, 72, 76
shelter, 46
shock, 60
short term memory, 22
short-term, 70
side effects, 32, 33, 52, 61, 67, 70, 77
signs, 13
sites, 29, 88
skills, 3, 7, 29, 41, 51, 55, 56, 65, 68, 69, 70, 72, 76, 78, 81, 82, 84
skills training, 69
skin, 10, 58, 77, 78
skin cancer, 10
skits, 24
sleep, 58
smoke, 15
smokers, 15
smoking, 15
social class, 36
social cognitive theory, 118
social group, 71
social justice, 37
social security, 2
social services, 7, 37
social support, 21, 30, 63, 67, 71, 74, 89, 108, 113, 115, 123
social welfare, 36, 37
social work, ix, 1, 2, 3, 4, 6, 7, 20, 23, 24, 25, 28, 31, 34, 41, 49, 50, 51, 52, 53, 54, 57, 58, 63, 66, 69, 70, 72, 73, 77, 78, 79, 80, 81, 82, 88, 90, 91, 93, 94, 95, 96, 97, 122, 123, 124, 125
social workers, ix, 1, 2, 3, 4, 6, 7, 20, 23, 25, 31, 34, 41, 51, 52, 53, 54, 58, 63, 66, 70, 72, 78, 80, 81, 82, 88, 90, 91, 93, 94, 95, 96, 97, 124, 125
socialist, 37
socioeconomic, 9, 13, 44, 110, 111, 122
socioeconomic status, 9, 13, 44, 110
somatic complaints, 70
sores, 58, 78
sounds, 57, 76
South Asia, 13
Southeast Asia, 27
specialization, 90
spectrum, 56, 96
speech, 37
spine, 33
spiritual, 2, 3, 34, 59, 60, 61, 62, 63, 71, 82, 107, 120, 121
spirituality, 59, 60, 61, 62, 63, 71, 120, 121
sponsor, 87

spouse, 53, 62, 74
St. Louis, 124
stability, 37
stages, 6, 10, 19, 21, 23, 24, 31, 57, 62, 69, 75, 118
stakeholders, 38
standards, 6, 29, 38, 45, 107, 109
statistics, 11, 12, 13, 14, 24
steel mill, 37
stigma, 26, 30
stigmatized, 30
strain, 21, 29, 30, 78
strains, 18
strategies, 4, 25, 33, 38, 39, 50, 56, 72, 75, 81, 84, 89, 91, 96, 112, 113, 120
strength, 31, 33, 35, 59, 60, 61, 120, 125
stress, 29, 30, 69, 70, 74, 76, 111, 114
stressors, 57
stress-related, 70
students, 94
subgroups, 27, 44
subjective, 53
sub-Saharan Africa, 13
subsidies, 41
suffering, 21, 40, 43, 75, 84, 115
supervisor, 94
supplements, 49
support services, 70, 72, 74
surgery, 12, 14, 23, 24, 25, 30, 45, 49, 67, 74, 75, 77, 78, 96, 112, 121
surgical, 67, 121
surveillance, 5
survival, 3, 6, 10, 11, 12, 14, 15, 22, 23, 24, 27, 32, 34, 35, 43, 45, 51, 56, 57, 61, 75, 110, 111, 113, 119
survival rate, 10, 11, 12, 15, 23, 24, 27, 32, 43
surviving, 20, 22, 23
survivors, ix, 1, 2, 3, 4, 5, 20, 22, 25, 29, 30, 31, 32, 33, 34, 35, 41, 50, 51, 53, 54, 55, 56, 57, 59, 60, 63, 66, 68, 69, 70, 71, 72, 76, 78, 79, 81, 82, 84, 85, 87, 89, 90, 94, 96, 97, 107, 115, 117, 118, 119, 120, 122, 123, 124
susceptibility, 110
sustainability, 93, 94
swelling, 58, 77
Switzerland, 43
sympathy, 28
symptoms, 3, 18, 21, 31, 53, 54, 65, 68, 77, 78
syphilis, 19
systemic change, 89
systems, 2

T

tamoxifen, 19, 111

tangible, 50
targets, 58
taxes, 37
team members, 1, 34, 82
technology, 36
Technology Assessment, 125
telephone, 31, 69, 70, 89
tenure, 36
terminally ill, 34, 115, 116, 120
Texas, 25, 36, 87, 114
Theodore Roosevelt, 36, 37
therapy, 14, 15, 17, 18, 19, 26, 29, 33, 45, 52, 69, 75, 76, 110, 111, 118, 122, 123
thinking, 25, 53
threat, 95
threatened, 37
threatening, 24
threats, 35
time, 1, 6, 11, 12, 13, 17, 18, 22, 23, 29, 30, 31, 32, 34, 35, 36, 37, 38, 39, 41, 43, 45, 47, 49, 50, 51, 53, 54, 55, 56, 57, 59, 61, 65, 68, 70, 71, 72, 74, 75, 77, 78, 79, 80, 81, 82, 83, 91, 94, 96, 105, 118
time frame, 34
tin, 58
tissue, 11, 23
toughness, 28
toxic, 22
tracking, 27
tradition, 7
training, 1, 2, 5, 7, 34, 35, 36, 69, 82, 84, 88, 94, 95, 107, 125
training programs, 95
trajectory, 57, 69
transition, 26, 57, 70, 76
transport, 37
transportation, 4, 23, 47, 50, 51, 58, 60, 72, 95
travel, 29, 30, 49
treatable, 24
trend, 10, 11, 12, 72, 83
trial, 111, 118, 119, 122, 123
tribal, 27
tribes, 27
trust, 33, 87
trusts, 53
tubal ligation, 17
tumor, 11, 13, 23, 29, 66, 110
tumors, 15, 16, 17, 19, 21, 23, 24, 45

U

U.S. economy, 43
uncertainty, 26, 33, 37, 79
underinsured, 40, 44, 47, 117
underreported, 68

unemployment, 24, 37
unemployment rate, 24
uninsured, 12, 14, 24, 43, 44, 45, 47
unions, 38
United States, vii, 9, 13, 14, 15, 35, 36, 40, 84, 109,
    113, 116
urban areas, 24, 51
urbanization, 35
US Department of Health and Human Services, 113
uterine cancer, 11, 12, 14, 16, 18, 26, 29
uterus, 10, 11, 14, 18, 19

V

vaccine, 19, 110
vagina, 10
Valdez, 114
validity, 62
values, 3, 7
variable, 3, 69
variables, 60
variation, 13, 117
vegetables, 14
venue, 77
Vietnamese, 25, 27
virus, 10, 19, 110
vocabulary, 32
vocational, 36
vocational training, 36
voice, 63, 83, 84, 91, 97
vomiting, 69
vulva, 10
vulvar, 10, 12, 15, 18, 19

W

wages, 46
war, 36
water, 37
web, 77, 87, 88, 91, 109, 113
web service, 77
websites, 87, 90, 91
weight gain, 52
weight management, 89
Weinberg, 123
welfare, 36
wellbeing, 79
well-being, 3, 7, 36, 56, 57, 61, 63, 68, 70, 72, 82,
    107
wellness, 1, 4, 71, 91
Western Europe, 13, 84
White House, 36
white women, 12, 24
Wisconsin, 112
wisdom, 124
work environment, 36
workers, 1, 2, 6, 7, 34, 36, 37, 41, 53, 58, 63, 68, 80,
    81, 90, 91, 93, 94, 95, 96, 97, 112
working conditions, 36
World Health Organization, 52
 worry, 26, 58, 61

Y

young women, 21